GET
HEALTHY
THROUGH
DETOX
AND FASTING

GET HEALTHY
THROUGH DETOX AND FASTING

DON COLBERT, MD

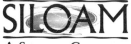

A STRANG COMPANY

Most STRANG COMMUNICATIONS/CHARISMA HOUSE/SILOAM/REALMS/
FRONTLINE products are available at special quantity discounts for bulk pur-
chase for sales promotions, premiums, fund-raising, and educational needs.
For details, write Strang Communications/Charisma House/Siloam/Realms/
FrontLine, 600 Rinehart Road, Lake Mary, Florida 32746, or telephone (407)
333-0600.

GET HEALTHY THROUGH DETOX AND FASTING by Don Colbert, MD
Published by Siloam
A Strang Company
600 Rinehart Road
Lake Mary, Florida 32746
www.siloam.com

Unless otherwise noted, all Scripture quotations are from the New King
James Version of the Bible. Copyright © 1979, 1980, 1982 by Thomas Nelson,
Inc., publishers. Used by permission.

Scripture quotations marked NIV are from the Holy Bible, New International
Version. Copyright © 1973, 1978, 1984, International Bible Society. Used by
permission.

Scripture quotations marked NLT are from the Holy Bible, New Living
Translation, copyright © 1996. Used by permission of Tyndale House
Publishers, Inc., Wheaton, IL 60189. All rights reserved.

Portions of this book appear in *The Seven Pillars of Health, Toxic Relief, Fasting
Made Easy,* and/or *The Bible Cure for Candida and Yeast Infections,* all by Don
Colbert, MD, and all published by Siloam.

Cover design by Judith McKittrick
Interior design by Terry Clifton

Library of Congress Cataloging-in-Publication Data

Colbert, Don.
  Get healthy through detox and fasting / Don Colbert.
      p. cm.
  Includes bibliographical references and index.
  ISBN 1-59185-961-1 (trade paper)
  1. Detoxification (Health) 2. Fasting. I. Title.
RA784.5.C65 2006
613--dc22

2006015284

06 07 08 09 10 — 987654321
Printed in the United States of America

CONTENTS

INTRODUCTION

Even though you may have never fasted in your life, something caused you to pick up this book. Something in you is drawing you to the idea of fasting and detoxifying your body of the toxins we face in today's world.

Maybe you are experiencing some of the physical symptoms of your toxic environment. You may have recognized your need for a healthier lifestyle and may be making choices to eliminate junk food and harmful chemicals from your life. Perhaps you are seeking a greater awareness of God's presence in your life and are searching for a spiritual discipline you can embrace.

We live in a dangerously toxic world. Deaths related to our toxic diet and lifestyle account for most deaths in America, including those from heart disease, cancer, strokes, diabetes, and obesity. Many of these diseases, and others, are caused by a buildup of toxins that overwhelm the body's vital organs and other systems, creating an array of distressing symptoms. Do you recognize any of these symptoms?

- Fatigue
- Memory loss
- Premature aging
- Skin disorders
- Arthritis
- Hormone imbalances
- Anxiety
- Emotional disorders
- Cancer
- Heart disease

After years as a medical practitioner and family physician, I'm convinced there is a better way. Not only can you prevent chronic illness and poor health due to toxicity, but also if you are suffering from some of these symptoms, you may even be able to turn your situation completely around.

In this book I am presenting you with a twenty-eight-day fasting program. If you will make a commitment to follow my plan, you will see benefits and results that will start you on the path to better health.

It will also be important for you to establish a new health-first lifestyle plan to follow from Day 29 through your future. I will give you some important guidelines for making choices that will give you the information and wisdom you need to be healthier and to eliminate some of the dangerous toxins that cause poor health.

This twenty-eight-day cleansing, detoxifying fast is designed to restore you to health—body, mind, and spirit. So, if you have been suffering from a toxic overload, you are ready to begin my twenty-eight-day plan. It is divided into two sections:

1. The twenty-one-day partial fast (you can adapt this to a Daniel fast if desired)

2. The seven-day detoxification juice fast

Fasting can improve your health physically and spiritually. Decide to begin my fasting program *today!* You will be glad you made that decision.

GET
HEALTHY

CHAPTER 1

I Live in a World Filled With Toxins

We live in a toxic world—one that is taking a heavy toll upon your body every day, whether you know it or not. Technological advances since the Industrial Revolution have resulted in dangerous chemicals and pollutants finding their way into our streams, soil, and air—toxins that enter and build up in our bodies, causing toxicity and, eventually, disease. Every day we are exposed to many types of toxins, and some are slowly accumulating in our bodies.

These toxins have changed our environment—around us in our world and within our bodies. For example, at this moment:

- Practically everyone has lead stored their bones.[1]

- Small amounts of DDT or its metabolite DDE are usually found in your fatty tissues.[2]

- Chemicals in tap water are now a major problem in the United States due to pollution.

- In 1993, more than 1,672,127,735 pounds of toxic chemicals were released into our air.[3]

- Pesticides, have been linked to brain cancer, prostate cancer, leukemia, and lymphoma, and they are sprayed on our produce and are present in higher concentrations in fatty cuts of meat and high fat dairy products such as butters and cheese.

SICK AND TOXIC

Lead, a soft, malleable metal, is utilized in building materials, batteries, bullets, pottery glaze, and other products. Because of its long-term and widespread use, lead has affected our entire planet through airborne contamination. It has been found in areas as remote as the Arctic Ice Cap and in the New Guinea aborigines who live far away from any sources of lead exposure.

Lead, mercury, and other metals and chemicals that have polluted much of our water, food, and air are nonbiodegradable, meaning they do not easily break down to less harmful forms. And it isn't just our earth that finds it hard to break down these chemicals. It is also difficult for our bodies to detoxify or eliminate them efficiently. Many times we lack the enzymes required to metabolize them. Thus, these chemicals become stored in our bodies. It has been established that we have between five hundred to seven hundred times more lead in our bones than our ancestors did.[4]

If our earth is sick and toxic, then there is a very good chance that most of us will eventually be sick and toxic. Unfortunately, we are usually unable to smell, taste, see, or sense most of the toxic chemicals to which we are exposed on a daily basis. As a result, it becomes increasingly difficult to avoid exposure. If we do not cleanse our bodies of these poisons, we will eventually develop fatigue, chronic degenerative diseases, and maybe even cancer. Could all of these toxins in our environment be the reasons why one in seven women in the United States develop breast cancer and one in six men in the United States develop prostate cancer?[5]

TOXINS IN OUR AIR

Some of the air we breathe is polluted by exhaust from our cars, buses, trains, and planes, and by pollution from industrial sites, waste disposal, and more. Carbon monoxide makes up about half of our air pollutants. Most of this comes from fuel. This dangerous gas has been directly linked to heart disease.[6]

Heavy metals and other pollutants are emitted from smelting plants, oil refineries, and incinerators. Ozone is the main chemical offender in smog. It irritates the eyes as well as the respiratory tract. The smog and air pollution in some of our major cities are so high at times in the summer months that residents are warned against exercising outside. The air can become so thick with chemicals that at times it can be difficult to see.

We can live for weeks without food and days without water, but only minutes without air. If the air we are inhaling contains smog, chemicals, carbon monoxide, heavy metals, and other pollutants, then it passes into our noses, into our lungs, and on through our bloodstream. With each breath, toxic chemicals are actually being pumped by the heart to every cell in our bodies via the bloodstream.

TOXINS IN OUR FOOD AND LAND

Pesticides continue to be sprayed onto our land, subsequently making their way into our food supply, only to become stored in fatty tissues such as the brain, breasts, and the prostate gland. Every year approximately 1.2 billion pounds of pesticides and herbicides are sprayed on the crops in America that make up our food supply.[7] The farmers who work closely with these chemicals are at a greatly increased risk of developing certain cancers, especially brain cancer, prostate cancer, leukemia, and lymphoma.[8] Some of these dangerous substances are known to last for hundreds and even thousands of years before breaking down.

DDT is an extremely dangerous poison that was banned in 1972 due to its devastating effect on wildlife, causing multiple abnormalities in the eggshells of many birds and deformities of reproductive organs of many other animals.

Bald eagles, condors, alligators, and other animals developed deformities, and their populations decreased dramatically. Nevertheless, residues from DDT or its close relative DDE are still present in the bodies of practically all Americans.

Pesticides have been linked to a lower sperm count in men and to higher amounts of xenoestrogen in women. *Xenoestrogen* is a chemical counterfeit that fools the body into accepting it as genuine estrogen. This estrogen is more potent than the estrogen made by the ovaries. When this occurs, a woman's hormones can become severely imbalanced, leading to symptoms of PMS, fibrocystic breast diseases, and potentially endometriosis. It can even have a stimulating effect on breast cancer and endometrial cancer.[9]

> FACTOID:
> Organic produce and free-range organic meats are typically very low in pesticides.

No doubt you have tried to wash off a shiny red apple or a dark green cucumber, only to find that it was covered with a layer of waxy film that is nearly impossible to wash off. Growers do this on purpose. The wax keeps the produce from dehydrating by sealing in water and makes vegetables look bright, shiny, and healthy. Most of these waxes, however, contain powerful pesticides or fungicides that have been added to keep the food from spoiling. If you want to stay healthy, remove these waxes (see chapter eight for more information on how to do this), or buy organic produce that does not contain the waxes.

Because heavy concentrations of pesticides are usually found in animal feed, our meat supply ends up tainted with pesticides, too. Pesticide chemicals accumulate in the fatty tissues of the animals we eat. When we bite into a fatty piece of steak, a greasy hamburger, sausages, bacon, butter, and cream, we are ingesting even more pesticide residues. Our bodies are designed to eliminate the toxins we eat. But when pesticides are not broken down and eliminated from the body, they become stored in its fatty tissues.

Pesticides are easily absorbed into the body through contact with the skin, by breathing them into the lungs, and by ingesting them through the mouth. Even though the body is designed to eliminate such dangerous poisons, the sheer amount of them that we encounter daily is far more than our bodies were ever designed to deal with. Therefore, pesticides, their metabolites, and other dangerous toxins eventually build up in our bodies over time. And the greater the buildup, the more difficult it becomes for the body to eliminate them. When such a residue of pesticides builds up in the body, we can begin to experience the following symptoms or diseases:

- Memory loss
- Depression
- Anxiety
- Psychosis
- Other forms of mental illness
- Parkinson's and other neurodegenerative diseases
- Possibly hormone-sensitive cancers such as breast, ovarian, uterine, and prostate cancer
- Fibromyalgia
- Multiple chemical sensitivity
- Allergies
- Fatigue
- Autoimmune diseases

TOXINS IN OUR WATER

Most chemicals that have been emitted into our air, sprayed on our farmlands, or dumped in our landfills will eventually end up in our water. Rains wash these chemicals out of the air and off our land into our lakes and rivers.

Nitrates from pesticides, herbicides, and fertilizers eventually end up in underground aquifers. The toxins gathered in chemical waste sites and dump sites, including landfills, can also eventually seep into our water supplies and contaminate them. Even underground storage tanks that hold gasoline can leak into the ground water. Rainstorms can actually wash these toxic chemicals into streams and larger bodies of water. Sooner or later, they may find their way into our drinking water supply.

Ground water supplies drinking water for approximately half of the people in America. Often municipalities treat ground water with aluminum to remove organic material, and traces of aluminum remain in the drinking water.

Most cities also add fluoride to the water. Fluoride partially inhibits approximately one hundred enzymes in the body. It interferes with vitamin and mineral functions and is linked to calcium deposits and arthritis.

Chlorine is also added to the water to kill microorganisms. Chlorine can also combine with organic materials to form trihalomethanes, which are cancer-promoting substances. We actually increase our risk of developing bladder and rectal cancer by drinking chlorinated tap water. In fact, the risk increases as our intake of chlorinated water increases.

Although chlorine kills most bacteria, it does not kill viruses and parasites. Parasites include helminths (worms), arthropods (ticks, mites, and other bugs), and protozoa such as amoeba, *giardia*, and *cryptosporidium*. Giardia is one of the major causes of diarrhea in day-care centers and contaminates many of the lakes and streams in America. It may be showing up in water supplies more often than we think. An outbreak of the microorganism *cryptosporidium* in Milwaukee's water supply in 1993 killed more than one hundred people and sickened another four hundred thousand.[10] Some observers believe that certain outbreaks of intestinal flu may actually be caused by such microorganisms in tap water.

INDOOR AIR POLLUTION

Indoor air pollution is often even more dangerous to your health than what you inhale outside. Most people spend about 90 percent of their time inside homes, office buildings, restaurants, factories, and school buildings. Indoor toxins, chemicals, and bacteria get trapped and circulated throughout the heating and air conditioning systems of these structures and may create a much greater health risk.

Today's buildings are much more airtight and well insulated than they were years ago, making them vaults for germs, bacteria, and chemical toxins. New buildings are the worst. Building materials emit gasses into the air through a process known as "out-gassing." New carpets release formaldehyde. Paints release solvents such as toluene and formaldehyde, and furniture made from pressed wood releases formaldehyde into the air as well. Additionally, out-gassing may also occur from fabrics, couches, curtains, carpet padding, glues, and more.

High amounts of volatile organic compounds can also be found in offices. These compounds are emitted from copying machines, laser printers, computers, and other office equipment. They cause headaches; itchy, red, and watery eyes; sore throats; dizziness; nausea; and concentration problems.

Airborne mold, bacteria, and the poisons given off by yeast can also cause pollution indoors. Many, if not most, air conditioning units and heating systems contain some amount of mold. The spores from that mold can travel throughout a building. Mold grows wherever dampness is found, which makes air conditioning units incubators for it. Damp homes not only breed mold, but they also breed dust mites. Dust mites are the most common airborne allergy.

Another powerful offender is cigarette smoke. The smoke from a burning cigarette as it sits lit in an ashtray contains a higher toxic concentration of gasses than what the smoker actually inhales.[11] Secondhand cigarette smoke contains cadmium, cyanide, lead, arsenic, tars, radioactive material, dioxin (which is a toxic pesticide), carbon monoxide, hydrogen cyanide, nitrogen oxides, nicotine, sulfur oxides, and about four thousand other chemicals.

THE DANGERS OF SOLVENTS

Solvents, which are chemicals used in cleaning products, are everywhere. Solvents dissolve other materials that otherwise would not be soluble in water.

Solvents can injure the kidneys and liver. They can also depress the elaborate central nervous system of our bodies. Like pesticides, solvents are fat-soluble, which simply means that they are likely to be stored in our fatty tissues, including, of course, the brain, breasts, and prostate gland. Solvents have the ability to dissolve into the membranes of our cells, especially our fat cells, and accumulate there. Take a look at some common solvents and the problems they cause:

- Formaldehyde is commonly used to make drapes, carpet, particleboard, and even cosmetics. Formaldehyde exposure is associated with nasal cancer, nasopharyngeal cancer, and possibly even leukemia.[12] Exposure to formaldehyde can also cause asthma, chronic headaches, memory lapse, nose bleeds, eye irritation, and other conditions.

- Phenol is widely found in cleaning products such as Lysol and is used to make aspirin and sulfa drugs. Phenol is easily absorbed by the skin and can cause burns, numbness, wheezing, headaches, nausea, vomiting, and irritability.

- Benzene is a solvent used in making dyes and insecticides. Long-term exposure to benzene can cause leukemia.

- Toluene is similar to benzene and is used for making a variety of different glues and typewriter correction fluids. Elevated levels of toluene in the body are associated with arrhythmias of the heart as well as nerve damage.

- Vinyl chloride is used in the manufacture of PVC pipes and plastic food wrappers, and it has been linked to several types of cancers and sarcomas.

- PCBs, which were banned in 1977, have contaminated many of our lakes and streams and are associated with an increased risk of all types of cancer. One study showed significant increase in deaths from gastrointestinal tract cancers in men who were exposed to PCBs and excess risk of death from leukemia in women who were exposed.[13]

As you can see, even our cells, tissues, and organs are being bombarded with toxic chemicals from every direction. We are being exposed to pesticides, solvents, and other chemicals through our food, water, and environment every day.

But we are not hopeless. We do not need to sit passively by while our immune systems break down and diseases develop under the heavy burden. Detoxification is available. We can cleanse our bodies from years of accumulated toxins and their effects by learning to support the body's own elaborate system of detoxification.

CHAPTER 2

I Battle Toxins Within My Body

Even if you lived in a perfect, unspoiled environment with no chemicals or poisons, your body would still produce its own toxins. Your body creates many different toxins in an infinite variety of ways just to function.

In a perfect environment, dealing with your body's internal toxins would be a cinch for your liver and excretory system. But your liver, GI tract, organs, and tissues have been bombarded from without and within with far more poisons than they were ever designed to handle. Take a look at some of these toxic enemies:

- If you have had repeated bouts of antibiotics, or even a single bout of superantibiotics, then you could be at risk for developing an overgrowth of dangerous intestinal bacteria and yeast.

- Millions of french fries are being produced in our bodies every day and, if unchecked, will set the stage for cancer, heart disease, and a host of other potentially fatal diseases.

- Too many sugars, fats, processed foods, fast foods, and other devitalized foods are literally draining the life out of us as they constipate our bodies, introduce toxins, and drain us of our nutrient reserves.

- Fried foods, hydrogenated and partially hydrogenated fats, excessive amounts of polyunsaturated fats, and food sensitivities cause inflammation in the body. We now know that arthritis, autoimmune disease, asthma, cardiovascular disease, Alzheimer's disease, and most cancers are associated with excessive inflammation.

WHEN THE CURE CAUSES THE CRISIS

Without antibiotics we'd be in trouble. Infections that might have snuffed out a life a century ago are little more than a nuisance today. But we are just beginning to get a full picture of the toll that the overuse of antibiotics has taken on a generation of users.

Your intestines are filled with good bacteria, such as *lactobacillus acidophilus* and *bifidus*, which prevent the overgrowth of pathogenic bacteria (bad bacteria) in your intestinal tract. When you take antibiotics, many of your body's beneficial bacteria can be killed. Your good bacteria function like a fire wall to keep pathogenic bacteria and yeast in check. So when antibiotics throw off the balance, the bad bacteria and yeast may grow like a wildfire, out of control with nothing to slow them down or stop them.

Bad bacteria may produce endotoxins, which may be as toxic as almost any chemical pesticide or solvent that enters your body from outside. Overgrowth of bacteria in your small intestines can cause excessive fermentation, just like the fermentation that happens when you leave apple cider outside for too long. This fermentation process creates even more poisons, such as *indoles, skatols,* and *amines.*

Just like a biblical plague of locusts that ravaged ancient farmlands, yeast overgrowth causes damage to the intestinal lining. Candida albicans is a yeast that releases over eighty different toxins into the body. Some of the most toxic substances produced by candida albicans are acetaldehyde and ethanol, which is alcohol. For more information on this topic, refer to my book *The Bible Cure for Candida and Yeast Infections*.[1]

The Environmental Protection Agency (EPA) has concluded that acetaldehyde is probably a human carcinogen, based on studies of its effects on animals.[2] German factory workers at a plant that processed acetaldehyde were found to have a higher cancer rate than normal, according to a study by the International Agency for Research on Cancer (IARC) in 1985.[3] Acetaldehyde is also extremely toxic to the brain, even more so than ethanol. It causes memory loss, depression, concentration problems, and severe fatigue.

When you consider the potential danger of having strong, devastating poisons created inside your body, you will recognize that the toxins within can do as much or even more damage than environmental toxins.

THE MOLECULAR WARFARE OF FREE RADICALS

While you are going about your daily business, a war is raging inside your body at the molecular level. Free radicals are similar to microscopic shrapnel, machine-gunning through the body, injuring cells and tissues throughout the day. Let me explain.

Picture an atom. It has a nucleus surrounded by electrons. The nucleus is positively charged, and the electrons are negatively charged. It looks something like the sun with the planets revolving around it.

When you are exposed to air pollution or radiation, when someone blows smoke in your face, or when you ingest alcohol or some other chemical or pesticide, the free radicals created by one of these toxins can pull one of the electrons out of orbit. When the atom, which is missing an electron, becomes unstable, it begins to grab electrons from other nearby molecules to replace it, causing chain reactions.

Free radicals are produced in the body, and in small numbers inside cells they are actually useful in activating many enzyme reactions and biological reactions. However, toxins such as air pollution, cigarette smoke, pesticides, solvents, and heavy metals cause the production of excessive amounts of free radicals, causing damage to cells, tissues, and organs.

Each of your body's trillions of cells has a protective wrapping around it made of lipids or "fatty" cell membranes. But free radicals, like wrecking balls, can start ricocheting off the cell membranes—eventually damaging intracellular structures such as the mitochondria and nucleus.

When free radicals begin a chain reaction, they must be stopped quickly. Antioxidants rush to the rescue instantly to quench the free-radical fire of activity. There are literally hundreds of different compounds that function as antioxidants. Many are found in foods and supplements, and others are naturally produced by the body. Many free radicals occur with normal metabolic processes in all cells in the body. Internal antioxidants such as superoxide dismutase, glutathione peroxidase, and catalase work as antioxidants, controlling free-radical production.

But problems occur when the level of free-radical activity gets out of control. When the body is overburdened with free radicals from air pollution, pesticides, solvents, cigarette smoke, fried foods, and polyunsaturated fats in our diet, then excessive amounts of free radicals ravage our cells. They can actually cause the breakdown of the fats in the cell membranes, ravage the proteins and enzymes, and then eventually damage DNA, actually causing mutations. These mutations may result in cancer.

A STRATEGY FOR WINNING THE WAR AGAINST TOXINS

You may feel overwhelmed by the monumental battle your cells, tissues, and organs are faced with each day. As you look in the mirror, you may even see some of the results of this war: premature aging, sickness, chronic fatigue, arthritis, cancer, heart disease, and so much more.

The good news is that you don't have to sit by passively while your God-given entitlement to good health is stolen right out from under your nose. Your body is designed with an incredible system of defense that keeps you healthy even under extreme circumstances—and you never have to give it a second thought. But when the battle becomes overwhelming, when toxins pile up inside you over time, your liver and excretory system may eventually become overburdened. They simply cannot keep up.

However, you can choose to step in and even the score. By undergoing my twenty-eight-day program of detoxification outlined in section three of this book, you can cleanse your body from a lifetime of toxins and discover the health and vitality that come with internal cleansing. You will simply be amazed at how much better you will feel after freeing your body of its toxic burden.

FACTOID:

Your mother may have taught you that the best vitamins are found in the skin of the potato—but so are the pesticides. Don't eat the potato skins unless you use organically grown potatoes.

In my practice, I have encouraged many of my chronically ill patients to undergo detoxification. The results have been astonishing. Heart disease, diabetes, hypertension, arthritis, chronic fatigue, and many other serious diseases are being absolutely reversed as my patients cleanse their own bodies from toxins. Your health will improve dramatically once those toxins are removed rather than circulated to other areas of the body. Not only will you feel better and live longer, but also you will actually look better, too.

YOUR PROGRAM FOR DETOXIFICATION

Here's an overview of my twenty-eight-day fasting program:

- You will start by undergoing a three-week partial fast to strengthen and support your liver and improve your elimination through the GI tract.

- Then you will go on a juice fast for seven days. You may need to be monitored by your doctor for this period of time. If you cannot fast for seven days, you will see tremendous results by fasting only one or two days.

- You will follow my four-day guidelines for breaking your fast. (Note: I would recommend that you go back on the special diet for your liver and GI tract for another two weeks after you complete my twenty-eight-day fasting program.

As you go through this fasting program, you will discover renewed energy, rejuvenated health, and a fresh, glowing sense of vitality that will absolutely astonish you.

However, my twenty-eight-day fasting program is only one part of a two-pronged solution for dealing with toxins on a regular basis. The second part is the importance of making lifestyle changes and establishing a plan to fast periodically in order to continue to cleanse and maintain your health. In order for you to understand how important it is for you to do both parts of this program, I want you to face the terrible truth about the American diet.

CHAPTER 3

I Need to Face the Truth About the American Diet

Most of America's health problems today are caused by dietary abuses. Elizabeth Frazao of the U. S. Department of Agriculture (USDA) reported that poor eating habits are linked to more than half of the deaths in the United States.

> Diet is a significant factor in the risk of coronary heart disease (CHD), certain types of cancer, and stroke—the three leading causes of death in the United States, and responsible for over half of all deaths in 1994. Diet also plays a major role in the development of diabetes (the seventh leading cause of death), hypertension, and obesity. These six health conditions incur considerable medical expenses, lost work, disability, and premature deaths— much of it unnecessary, since a significant proportion of these conditions is believed to be preventable through improved diets.[1]

There are many ways we abuse our bodies through our poor eating habits, but here are a few of the major abusers in our diets:

- The average American consumes 150 pounds of sugar per year. That's the equivalent of about one to two teaspoons of sugar per hour![2]

- Processed foods are grossly deficient in nutrients and contain food additives, sweeteners, flavorings, coloring agents, preservatives, bleaching agents, emulsifiers, texturizers, humectants, acids, alkalis, buffers, and other chemicals. Such foods provide loads of calories with little nutrition.

- Our soil has been robbed of important minerals and nutrients; therefore, the food it produces is nutritionally poor.

- The fat we eat, including saturated fats and hydrogenated fats, overtax our bodies with thick, sludgelike, yellowish-brown material that encrusts the inside of our arteries, forms plaque, fattens our bodies, elevates our cholesterol, forms stones in our gallbladders, weakens our immune system, and shortens our lives.

- Fast foods, fried foods, and eating far too much meat while denying our bodies healthful fruits and vegetables are ways in which we abuse our bodies through our diets.

It's easy to see why we're overfed and undernourished. We gorge ourselves with increasing amounts of food to respond to our bodies' cravings for nutrition. After we've eaten, our bodies, even though under a heavy burden of calories, still realize that they never received the nutrients they needed. So our brains send more signals, triggering hunger, which is interpreted by us as the need or desire for even more food. We end up spiraling down into a vicious cycle of overfeeding with empty foods, craving more nutrition and overfeeding again with even more empty, processed, devitalized, sugary foods.

The end result is ever-expanding waistlines, thighs, and buttocks. We get fatter and fatter, forcing our bodies to groan under the burden of extra pounds. But in terms of actual nourishment, we give our bodies less and less.

We may be actually starving from a nutritional standpoint while at the same time becoming grossly obese. The end result of this merciless abuse of our bodies is disease and death. Sadly, we really are digging our graves with our forks and knives!

As a result of our overindulgences we have an epidemic of heart disease, atherosclerosis, hypertension, diabetes, cancer, allergies, obesity, arthritis, osteoporosis, and a host of other painful and debilitating degenerative diseases.

JUNK FOOD OVERLOAD

Americans have been duped into believing that we can continued to exist on junk food day by day and simply add a multivitamin—or a multitude of vitamins—a day to protect ourselves from whatever we have eaten while maintaining excellent health. Taking vitamins and other nutrients while continuing to eat poorly is similar to adding small amounts of oil to keep a car's oil level in normal range, but never changing the oil or oil filter while continuing to drive it.

Over the years as I have treated people with degenerative diseases, I have noticed a pattern. Most of these individuals aren't underfed. In fact, most of them are big overeaters. They eat plenty—but they eat all the wrong things. They are overfed and yet completely undernourished. This is particularly true of most people with obesity, cardiovascular diseases, arthritis, type 2 diabetes, migraine headaches, a host of different allergic conditions, psoriasis, rheumatoid arthritis, and lupus. In fact, to some degree, it appears to apply to nearly all degenerative diseases.

For many of these people, medications won't help. Nor can taking vitamins and nutrients eliminate the cause of these diseases. That's because it is not lack that causes many of these diseases—it is eating too much of the wrong foods.

One of the main causes of these degenerative diseases is overconsumption of sugary, fatty, starchy, and high-protein foods—foods that have been processed, fried, and further devitalized. These people were taking in enormous amounts of empty, fattening calories, but they were not nourishing their bodies.

Taking supplements such as a comprehensive multivitamin with minerals, antioxidants, and so forth is important. However, it is much more important to eliminate (or significantly reduce) consumption of fat, sugar, and processed foods and to eat more fruits, vegetables, whole grains, nuts, seeds, and other whole foods.

Overnutrition is many times worse than undernutrition. In fact, animal studies have shown that getting too few calories, which is technically called *calorie restriction*, can actually increase longevity.[3] Although I do recommend calorie restriction for some diseases, such as type 2 diabetes and obesity, I believe that as a nation we need to work harder at eating in a way that keeps us within a healthy weight range.

STOP AND THINK ABOUT HOW YOU EAT

Our prosperity as a nation has come at a price. After years of overeating and overindulgence, we are experiencing an epidemic of degenerative diseases.

Most of us eat a standard American diet. That means lots of fat, sugar, and highly refined wheat products, including white bread, crackers, bagels, pasta, and cereals. Add other processed food, such as potato chips, corn chips, and white rice. Don't forget the fatty meats like T-bone steaks, ribs, bacon, and pork chops. Now, top it all off with a large amount of saturated fat, hydrogenated fat, and processed vegetable fat, such as salad dressing, peanut butter, most cooking oils, and mayonnaise. It's no wonder we have an epidemic of heart disease, cancer, diabetes, and arthritis, as well as many other degenerative diseases.

Now for dessert. What could be more American than apple pie? Nevertheless, the absolute worst foods—and all-time American favorites—contain tons of sugar and hydrogenated fat. These include many baked goods, such as cupcakes, cookies, pies, pastries, fudge, and brownies—and don't forget the doughnuts and candy bars.

We didn't always eat this way. Former generations were some of the healthiest on the planet. As an agrarian culture, many of our grandparents lived much closer to the land. But today, our lifestyle is much too stressed and fast-paced, and as a result, our diet suffers.

CHANGE THE WAY YOU THINK

Most of us have grown up eating the American diet and feeling pretty good about it. But to live healthier, longer lives, we must rethink what we have been taught about food—before it's too late.

We begin to change our thinking by changing the *why* of eating. *Just why do you eat?* Do you eat because something tastes good and your flesh is craving it, or because you are stressed, anxious, lonely, or depressed? Or do you eat because you are providing your body with fuel to run? For most Americans, eating has become more of a recreation than a daily necessity based upon nutritional wisdom.

Now, I'm not trying to suggest that meals shouldn't be enjoyed. God created all things for us to enjoy, and eating was one of those things. But when our dietary choices, which were designed to nourish and sustain our bodies, actually begin to make us ill, then we must change the way we think.

Hippocrates, the father of medicine, said, "Our food should be our medicine, and our medicine should be our food." In other words, what we eat should be so good for us that it actually heals and restores our bodies. What a difference from the average American mind-set about eating!

Start thinking about more than just taste and pleasure when you eat. Begin to eat for your health's sake!

So, here's your new set of priorities: health first, taste and pleasure second. I guarantee that once you begin to satisfy the true need of your body—the need for genuine nourishment—you will begin to enjoy your food much more.

Right now, before you even begin to follow my twenty-eight-day fasting program, determine that the minute the twenty-eight days is over, you will start following a health-first eating lifestyle. Before you begin the fasting program, go through your cupboards, pantry, refrigerator, and freezer and eliminate or drastically reduce fried foods (chips, french fries, chicken nuggets, etc.), processed foods (any food that man has tampered with and packaged, such as instant oatmeal, instant rice, most cereals, etc.), processed vegetable fats, saturated fats, hydrogenated and partially hydrogenated fats, and sugary foods. Prepare a grocery list now for your new health-first eating plan, and stock your pantry in preparation for Day 29! Determine to avoid fatty cuts of meats and to select smaller portions of the leanest meats, including free-range or organic chicken or turkey breast and free-range or organic beef such as extra-lean ground round, tenderloin, and filet.

YOUR HEALTH-FIRST FIVE-ALIVE PLAN

In your new health-first eating plan, you will want to eat at least five servings of living, organic vegetables and fruits every day. (By *living*, I mean that the naturally occurring nutrients in the plants have not been altered or depleted through processing, packaging, storage, or preparation.) As of 2005, the recommendation of the USDA is five to thirteen servings of fruits and vegetables per day.[4] That means fruits and vegetables should make up a large percentage of your diet.

LIMIT MEATS

The Bible does not recommend vegetarianism, so neither do I. Adam and Eve were vegetarians in the Garden of Eden, and some prophets, such as John the Baptist, Samson, Samuel, and others who had taken Nazirite vows, were vegetarians. Still, Jesus Christ was not.

Nevertheless, most Americans eat far too much meat. I recommend that women eat only 2 to 3 ounces of lean, free-range meat, once or twice daily. Men, limit meats to only 4 ounces of lean, free-range meat, once or twice daily. And I always recommend chewing every bite thirty times.

AVOID HIGH-PROTEIN DIETS

More and more people are going on high-protein diets such as the Atkin's diet. Yes, they are losing weight. But the long-term effects of this diet can be very dangerous and may lead to many degenerative diseases.

If you are on this diet, limit your protein portions to no more than 4 ounces for men and 3 ounces for women once or twice a day. For more information on this subject, refer to my book *What You Don't Know May Be Killing You.*[5]

IN CONCLUSION

If you see yourself in this chapter, be encouraged. Even if you have spent a lifetime digging your own grave with your fork and knife, it's never too late to change. You will make many choices about your destiny by what you choose to eat. Choose now to reap health, happiness, and a long life. You hold the key to your own future health.

Before we begin the twenty-eight-day fasting program, let's look at what I believe is the single most effective answer to overnourishment—fasting! More than anything else, fasting is a dynamic key to cleansing your body from a lifelong collection of toxins, reversing overnourishment and the diseases it brings, and ensuring a wonderful future of renewed energy, vitality, longevity, and blessed health.

CHAPTER 4

There Are Many Benefits to Fasting

Fasting is not new. In fact, it has been around since before Moses. Many methods of fasting exist, as well as many attitudes about fasting. As a doctor, I have been able to look closely at the various popular methods of fasting. Some of them are good, while others can be downright dangerous. Fasting is often thought of as taking nothing by mouth. Technically speaking, this is true, but it's not the type of fasting I suggest for detoxification. I consider total fasting—not eating or drinking anything—to be unsafe. Your body must always have at least two quarts of water a day to sustain your life, for you can only live for a few days without water. Although there are many ways to fast, the kind of fast that will bring about the optimum health benefits described in this book is the combination of a partial fast and juice fast. This type of fasting provides fantastic health benefits to your body, mind, and spirit. For example:

- Fasting gives a restorative rest to your digestive tract.

- Fasting helps the body's designed healing processes to automatically work by giving them a chance to rest from other activities.

- This rest from "digestion as usual" in turn allows your overburdened liver to catch up with its task of detoxification.

- Your blood and lymphatic system also receive needed cleansing of toxic buildup through fasting.

- Fasting allows your other digestive organs, including the stomach, pancreas, intestines, and gallbladder, a much deserved rest, which allows your cells time to heal, repair, and be strengthened.

A powerful, natural way to bring relief to your body from the burden of excess toxicity, fasting is also a safe way to heal and prevent degenerative diseases. As you can see from the list above, the primary way that fasting allows your body to heal is by giving it a rest.

THE PRINCIPLE OF REST

As with all living things, you need to rest. Sleeping is not the only kind of rest you need. Your digestive system and other organs need a rest from their work as well. This understanding of the human need for rest is not new to mankind. God introduced the principle of a "Sabbath rest" to His ancient Jewish nation. It is one of the Ten Commandments: "Remember the Sabbath day, to keep it holy" (Exod. 20:8). Israel was given specific instructions regarding this divine command to work six days and to rest on the seventh day of each week. This principle of rest was important as well to their agricultural system. The Israelites were commanded to allow their fields to lie fallow every seventh year in order to give the soil the "rest" it needed to reestablish its own mineral and nutrient content. (See Leviticus 25:1–7.)

Today, this biblical agricultural principle of resting the soil has been ignored by virtually all modern farmers. As a result, the soil has become depleted of some of the minerals and other nutrients that our bodies crave for health. And chemical fertilizers do not succeed in giving us the abundant mineral content of healthy soil.

It is interesting to note that in the animal kingdom, it is a natural habit to seek rest and to abstain from food, especially when the animal is sick or injured. A sick animal refuses to eat and finds a place to rest where it can lap up water and be safe. Some animals hibernate, resting for an entire season without eating.

Rest is also a powerful principle of healing for the human body and psyche. Every night as you sleep, you are providing refreshing rest for your mind and body, which aids health in a tremendous way. Sleep deprivation is a commonly known form of torture, emphasizing the fact of our innate need for rest.

Fasting may be considered an "internal" rest for the body, allowing it to restore vitality and energy to vital organs by activating the marvelous self-cleansing system with which it is designed.

ENJOYING THE PHYSICAL BENEFITS OF FASTING

To help convince you of the potentially healing benefits of fasting, let me explain briefly the marvelous natural detoxification system God designed for your body. Proper understanding of the innate healing power resident in your body will help you appreciate the phenomenal benefits of fasting.

Your body's natural detox system

The hardest working organ in the body is the liver. Weighing about five pounds, it is also the largest single organ in the body, about the size of a football. It is designed to perform about five hundred functions for the health of the body. Let's look at them:

1. Filtering your blood to remove toxins such as viruses, bacteria, and yeast
2. Storing vitamins, minerals, and carbohydrates
3. Processing fats, proteins, and carbohydrates
4. Producing bile to break down fats for digestion
5. Breaking down and detoxifying the body of hormones, chemicals, toxins, and metabolic waste

In just one minute your liver can filter about two quarts of the five quarts of blood your body contains. To appreciate the magnitude of this feat, you could compare your liver to the filter in a swimming pool. The filter would need to clean half of the pool's water every minute to keep up with what your liver can do. What an incredibly powerful filter your liver is! If it is working efficiently, it can filter out 99 percent of the bacteria and other toxins in your blood before sending the cleansed blood back into circulation.

Every day your liver produces about a quart of bile, which helps to digest dietary fats, breaking them down into a form that can be used as fuel for the body. The bile also functions to eliminate toxins from your body, flushing them out through your colon. For a more complete discussion of these important detoxifying functions of your liver, please read my book *Toxic Relief.*[1]

Unfortunately, when this natural filter gets overwhelmed with toxins, it cannot function well, much as a dirty air filter in your car cannot remove dirt from the air. Your liver may get overloaded with toxins from our food and water; from food allergies; from parasites; from toxins in the air, home, or workplace; and from free radicals produced internally in the liver by the detoxification process itself. Like dust and dirt that accumulate in your air filter, these toxins make the liver work too hard; eventually, it cannot function efficiently. That is why fasting becomes important, to allow the liver to rest and be able to catch up with its cleansing duties.

Some signs of liver toxicity include the following:

- Pallid skin
- A coated tongue
- Bad breath
- Skin rashes
- Poor skin tone
- Itchy, weepy, swollen, and red eyes
- Yellow discoloration of the eyes

- Body odor
- Itchy skin
- Altered or bitter taste in your mouth

It is vital that you have a healthy liver in order to be healthy. You should do everything you can to keep this champion prizefighter healthy and working at peak efficiency. Fasting is a wonderful way to improve the efficiency of your detoxification system. The first twenty-one days of the fasting program presented in section three are designed to provide you with a nutritional program to support and strengthen your liver.

Restoring a healthy GI tract

Have you ever worked on a computer that was overloaded with files, programs, and unnecessary junk? If so, you realize that as a result of being overloaded, your computer works slower and slower, perhaps finally giving up the ghost and refusing to work altogether. Your GI tract can suffer a shutdown in a similar way as a result of overloading it with too much junk food. When people consistently overeat or consume an inadequate amount of fiber, they are placing an enormous strain on their GI tract. Even worse, many people do their overeating late at night, which does not allow the GI tract to rest even when you go to bed; it is still digesting all that "food."

The small intestine has been designed for several major functions to maintain your health.

- It acts as an organ of digestion and absorption of nutrients to fuel your body's energy level.

- It becomes a protective barrier to keep your body from absorbing toxic materials and other undesirable matter, such as large molecules of undigested food.

- It allows ready absorption of needed nutrients such as *triglycerides* from the digestion of fats, *sugars* from the digestion of carbohydrates, *amino acids* and *di-* and *tri-peptides* from the digestion of proteins—all vital compounds needed to ensure your health.

- It also seals out toxins, heavy metals, undigested bits of food, and other matter that could cause your body harm.

In chapter five, we will discuss the specific physical conditions that can be reversed and prevented through regular fasting, but here are some of the general benefits your body will enjoy.

Increasing energy and mental clarity

A wonderful benefit of cleansing the body through proper fasting is increased energy levels. Cellular toxins and free radicals impair the mitochondria (the energy factories in each cell), hindering them from producing energy effectively. As a result, you may suffer fatigue, irritability, and lethargy. But when you fast, you allow your cells to shed many toxins so they can again produce the energy you need. Along with increased energy, you will most likely enjoy improved mental functioning as your body cleanses, repairs, and rejuvenates every organ, including your brain.

Boosting your immune system

Short-term fasting will also boost your immune system, which will help prevent disease and illness and give you a longer life. Along with an improved quality of life, you will discover that fasting even makes you look better. Your skin will eventually become clearer, giving you a radiance you have not known since your youth. The whites of your eyes will usually become clearer—they may even sparkle.

Restoring nature's delicate balance

When your body is too acidic, precious minerals are lost in the urine and cells become less permeable, which means they are unable to excrete waste products effectively. In a sense, your cells become constipated; they are full of waste and cannot eliminate it. As the cells become more and more toxic, free-radical activity increases, and the toxic overload continues to build until your body starts to deteriorate and degenerative diseases occur. However, fasting brings back the natural balance. It alkalinizes the tissues and raises the pH. This enables the cells to excrete toxins again and begins the process of detoxifying your body from head to toe.

Helping you lose weight

Not only does fasting free your body of disease-causing chemicals, but it will also free it of toxic fat. If you are over-weight, and even significantly obese, one of the truly wonderful and healthful benefits of partial fasting and juice fasting is that it can help bring your body back to the normal, healthy size that God intended. A regular, sensible fasting program can slim you down very quickly, and you will also experience the more important benefit of reducing the fatty areas in your body where dangerous toxins and chemicals were stored.

CAUTION: WHEN YOU SHOULD NOT FAST

There are health conditions and other situations that prohibit fasting for certain individuals. While the following list is not exhaustive, it does include some major conditions that prevent you from fasting. Please consult your physician before considering a fast, regardless of your state of health. However, if you have any of the following, DO NOT fast:

- Do not fast if you are pregnant or nursing.

- Do not fast if you are extremely debilitated or malnourished, such as patients with cancer,

AIDS, severe anemia, or any severe wasting conditions.

- Do not fast before or after surgery, since it may interfere with your ability to heal.

- Do not fast if you suffer from cardiac arrhythmia or congestive heart failure.

- Do not fast if you are struggling with mental illness, including schizophrenia, bipolar disorder, major depression, and severe anxiety.

- Do not fast if you suffer from severe liver or kidney disease.

- Do not fast if you are a type 1 diabetic.

- Do not fast if you are taking anti-inflammatory medications, aspirin, antidepressants, narcotics, chemotherapy, or diuretics. (Medications such as thyroid hormones and hormone replacement therapy are safe to take during a fast. Always consult your physician before fasting if you are taking any medication.)

- Do not fast if you are taking prednisone. You will need to first wean off this medication slowly under a doctor's supervision. (You may continue to take low doses of hypertension medications during a fast as long as you are monitored by a physician. However, this does not include diuretics.)

As a physician, I try to help wean my patients off most of their medications prior to supervising a fast for them. If your physician cannot wean you off your medications, then it may be safer to stay on the cleansing and detox fast outlined in chapter seven.

For any extended fast I recommend getting a checkup or physical exam by your doctor first. Have him or her do blood work and a baseline EKG. I normally perform a SMAC 24. This includes kidney function tests (including creatinine and BUN), electrolytes, liver function tests, blood sugar, cholesterol, and triglycerides. Along with the SMAC 24, I also perform a CBC, urinalysis (UA), and EKG. These tests should be performed prior to the fast.

During the fast, I will usually perform a SMAC 24 and urinalysis once or twice a week. During each office visit, tell your doctor if you are experiencing any severe weakness, fatigue, or light-headedness. Tell your doctor if you are having any irregular heartbeats. Again, if you develop an irregular heartbeat or pulse, you should be examined by your physician and should probably terminate the fast.

During a fast, it is critically important to make sure your blood potassium level remains in the normal range. Low potassium can cause dangerous arrhythmias of the heart and death. That's why it's critically important not to take diuretics on a fast. Juice fasting, however, supplies large amounts of potassium in the fresh-squeezed juices; therefore, it's very unlikely that you will develop low potassium while on the juice fast. Water fasts are more likely to cause low potassium levels. Commonly during a fast, the uric acid level is elevated. However, this is no cause for concern, since this is a normal response of the body to fasting. However, if you have gout, you will need to be monitored more closely by your physician and will need to drink adequate amounts of clean, pure water, not tap water.

Children under the age of eighteen should not follow a strict juice fast unless they are closely monitored by a physician.

REAP THE BENEFITS OF HEALTHY EATING

Whether physical conditions prevent you from fasting or not, there are steps everyone can take to improve intestinal health and establish a healthy eating plan. I recommend that, in addition to using the detoxification and fasting program presented in this book, you do the following:

- Always avoid overeating.

- Reinoculate the bowel with supplements containing friendly bacteria: *lactobacillus acidophilus* for the small intestines and *bifido* bacteria for the large intestine. These good bacteria can also help prevent damage to the lining of the GI tract, thus maintaining normal intestinal permeability.

- Refrain from excessive eating before bedtime.

- Determine to decrease the stress in your life, especially when eating, by choosing to eat in a relaxed, peaceful atmosphere.

- Stock your pantry with health-first items and eliminate processed, refined, devitalized foods.

Fasting and establishing healthy eating plans are the first two steps to help you feel and look better than you have in years. However, in order to keep your body detoxified from the harmful toxins in our world, you will have to fast repeatedly to detoxify the body and achieve vibrant health. Regular fasting is a healthy, biblical way to cleanse your body and soul. In the next section of this book, we will take a look at the benefits we can experience both physically and spiritually when we embark on a health-first lifestyle that incorporates regular fasting.

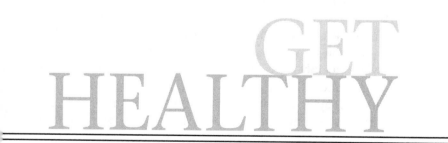

CHAPTER 5

Living a Healthier Life Through Regular Fasting

I am confident that as you embark on the fast outlined in this book, you will discover that your physical body is an amazing, natural detoxifier. No doubt you will reap many benefits during this detoxification program. But detoxification is more than a twenty-eight-day change; it is a lifestyle change.

In this toxic world, it takes more than a passive approach to health care to live long, healthy, active, disease-free lives. It takes wisdom. In the first section of this book I presented you with the wisdom I have gained as a medical doctor. As you continue to apply these truths in your future, you will reap the wonderful reward of renewed energy, vitality, and health.

The power of better health through detoxification is yours. I encourage you to pursue your own good health aggressively by looking carefully at your diet and lifestyle. Your own healthy future is in your hands! As you prepare for this short-term, twenty-eight-day fast, you also need to prepare for a long-term lifestyle change that puts health first.

As you begin to think about your new health-first lifestyle, remember that God created your body to quickly, cleanly, and efficiently deal with any toxin it may encounter. In this chapter I want to introduce you to some of the benefits to your physical body of including periods of regular fasting in your health-first lifestyle. The excessive buildup of toxins contributes to many physical diseases and conditions. Regular fasting is a way to eliminate these toxins and to restore your body to better health.

As you begin, consider the list of some of the diseases that are often directly linked to a buildup of toxins:

Food and environmental allergies	Abdominal bloating
Psoriasis	Belching
Lupus	Gas
Rheumatoid arthritis	Memory loss
Asthma	Chronic diarrhea
Headaches	Crohn's disease
Fatigue	Ulcerative colitis
Fibromyalgia	Atherosclerosis
Chronic back pain	Hypertension
Eczema, chronic acne, and other skin conditions	Obesity
Insomnia	Constipation
Depression	Angina
Irritable bowel syndrome	Multiple sclerosis
Decreased sex drive	Coronary artery disease
Menstrual problems	Cancer
	Mental illness
	Diabetes

Regular fasting holds amazing healing benefits to those of us who suffer illness and disease. From colds and flu to heart disease, regular fasting is a mighty key to healing the body. Let's look at some ways that regular fasting can be used to bring health and healing to a sick body.

FASTING FOR TYPE 2 DIABETES

If you have type 1 diabetes, you should not fast. However, fasting is extremely effective for most type 2 diabetics. Type 2 diabetics should not fast using fruits or vegetables that have a high glycemic index, such as carrot juice. Instead, you should fast using a well-balanced, high-fiber protein supplement.

(See Appendix B.) It is also critically important for diabetics to be on a low-glycemic diet and an aerobic exercise program. For more information on diabetes, see *The Bible Cure for Diabetes*.[1]

Because most individuals with type 2 diabetes also suffer from obesity, fasting is a great way to conquer your weight problems. But remember that fasting for too long can lower your metabolic rate and predispose you to gain even more weight. Short, frequent juice fasts—about three days out of every month—followed up with a healthy eating plan can bring obesity under control quickly and easily.

FASTING FOR CORONARY DISEASE

Fasting is very effective for the treatment of heart disease and peripheral vascular disease, which usually occurs in the legs. Peripheral vascular disease is simply a buildup of plaque or atherosclerosis, usually in the arteries of the lower extremities. Periodic fasting may help with plaque removal in the arteries.

While fasting, if you have significant coronary artery disease or peripheral vascular disease, you will find that your cholesterol levels will usually become more elevated on the fast. This happens because your body is in the process of breaking down plaque that is formed in the arteries, so don't be alarmed.

I always check the blood work before prescribing fasting for my patients. I'm always really encouraged when I see a dramatic elevation in cholesterol in those with coronary artery disease or peripheral vascular disease while fasting. I know that the fasting is doing its work and usually plaque is being broken down and removed while fasting.

FASTING FOR BENIGN TUMORS

Undergoing my twenty-eight-day fast may help to reduce the size of benign tumors. These include ovarian cysts, fibrocystic breast disease, lipomas, sebaceous cysts, and even uterine fibroids. If you have advanced cancer, you should not fast. But regular fasting will definitely help you to prevent cancer.

FASTING FOR CROHN'S DISEASE AND ULCERATIVE COLITIS

Fasting is very effective for patients with both Crohn's disease and ulcerative colitis. These diseases are usually associated with increased intestinal permeability, toxic overload on the liver, candida overgrowth, parasites, dysbiosis (bad bacteria), and numerous food allergies and sensitivities.

Many of my patients with Crohn's disease or ulcerative colitis are very sensitive to all dairy products, nightshades (including jalapeño peppers, potatoes, tomatoes, and eggplant), wheat products, and often yeast-containing products as well. These individuals are generally extremely sensitive to all forms of sugar. Simple sugars should therefore be totally eliminated from their diet.

Due to their sensitivity to sugar, these people do best on either a balanced rice protein supplement (see Appendix B) or on a water fast. Juice fasting with low-glycemic vegetable juices is also usually effective. However, juicing may aggravate the condition and lead to worsening of diarrhea.

Once your fast is over, continue eating rice products—primarily brown or wild rice, brown rice bread, and rice crackers. Slowly reintroduce a low-protein, primarily vegetarian diet into your health-first lifestyle similar to the first three weeks of the program. In addition, keep a good food diary to find out what foods cause food sensitivities, and avoid anything that irritates your GI tract.

FASTING FOR AUTOIMMUNE DISEASES

Autoimmune diseases are simply diseases in which the immune system attacks itself. A healthy immune system can tell the difference between normal cells and invader cells. However, in autoimmune diseases such as lupus and rheumatoid arthritis, the immune system gets confused. It actually produces antibodies that attack and inflame the body's own tissues. Eventually it can damage and even destroy the tissue.

Rheumatoid arthritis and lupus are autoimmune diseases that are often linked to altered intestinal permeability. This can also happen when you take too many antibiotics that decrease the numbers of friendly bacteria in the intestines or if your intestinal tract has been damaged by anti-inflammatory medications, aspirin, or food allergies.

Autoimmune disease can also be aggravated or caused by poor digestion and overconsumption of meats. Most Americans eat lots of meat and other animal proteins. Our bodies are not equipped to produce the amount of hydrochloric acid and digestive enzymes necessary to digest so much meat. Combine this with the load of stress that most of us live under, which further reduces the amount of the digestive juices such as hydrochloric acid and pancreatic enzymes, and it is no wonder we have an epidemic of bloating, gas, and indigestion!

We eat far too much protein for the amount of hydrochloric acid and digestive enzymes we produce. Therefore, our stomachs and intestines usually can't break down the proteins into the individual amino acids as well as they should. Incompletely digested proteins called *peptides* are formed. Peptides can be absorbed directly into the bloodstream if you have altered intestinal permeability. Your body may form antibodies to attack these foreign substances. Once again, the body may start to attack itself; if this happens, inflammation will occur.

Too much protein, poor digestion, and altered intestinal permeability are a recipe for autoimmune diseases such as rheumatoid arthritis and lupus. Such diseases are rare in countries such as Japan, China, and Africa where people eat mainly fruits, vegetables, and whole grains. But when these same people come to the United States and adopt our diet, they stand a greater risk of eventually developing autoimmune diseases.

Fasting is one of the most effective therapies for treating autoimmune diseases, but the earlier in the course of the disease, the better. Juice fasting is especially beneficial in autoimmune diseases. Nevertheless, some physicians have had outstanding results with water fasting. If you are going on a fast, especially a water fast, for an autoimmune disease, be sure you are carefully monitored by your physician. I do not recommend water fasts for individuals who are underweight.

If you have been taking prednisone or other steroid drugs, it is extremely important to wean off these medicines slowly, under medical supervision, prior to fasting. Be sure to watch for signs of adrenal suppression. They include severe weakness and fatigue, rapid heart rate, low blood sugar, and low blood pressure. It may take months to successfully wean off these medications.

After the fast, patients with autoimmune disease should decrease consumption of all animal proteins, dairy products, and eggs as a part of your health-first lifestyle. It may also be helpful to avoid wheat products and nightshades (such as tomatoes, potatoes, peppers, and eggplant). Instead, choose brown rice bread, rice crackers, spelt pasta, and other rice products.

FASTING FOR ALLERGIES AND ASTHMA

Juice fasting is extremely helpful if you have allergies or asthma. Your lungs, as well as your entire respiratory tract, are vitally important elimination organs for removing toxins. Fasting often removes many of the irritants and toxins that trigger airway hyperactivity.

Allergies—both airborne and food-related—will usually dramatically improve during a fast. Allergic symptoms are improved and sometimes completely disappear. However, it's important to be sure that you are not allergic to any of the juices or foods you will be consuming. Keep a food diary while you are on your fast. Use it to help you avoid anything that may trigger allergic symptoms or symptoms of asthma.

FASTING FOR PSORIASIS AND ECZEMA

I have found that many of my patients with psoriasis and/or eczema suffer from numerous food sensitivities. They usually have increased intestinal permeability and impaired liver detoxification.

It is critically important for those with psoriasis or eczema to fast with juices to which they are not allergic or to use a balanced rice protein supplement. (See Appendix B.) This is best done by having food allergy testing first or by choosing juices according to blood type. For more information on juices that are compatible with certain blood types, refer to my book *Toxic Relief.*

If you have psoriasis or eczema, you may also have yeast overgrowth in your intestinal tract. If you do have yeast overgrowth, parasites, or dysbiosis (bad bacteria), prior to fasting follow a candida diet for at least three months. For more information on candida and yeast overgrowth, refer to my book *The Bible Cure for Candida and Yeast Infections.*

If you find that you do not respond well to a juice fast, you can try a balanced rice protein fast (see Appendix B), which helps to detoxify the liver. This is an excellent fast for individuals with psoriasis, eczema, fibromyalgia, chronic fatigue, migraine headaches, multiple chemical sensitivities, and autoimmune diseases; it is also good for anyone with impaired detoxification capacity.

Water fasting can also be effective for psoriasis or eczema, but it must be closely monitored. If you decide to go on a water fast, supplement your fast with detoxifying teas such as dandelion and milk thistle tea.

Before going on any fast for psoriasis or eczema, follow the twenty-one-day liver support fast that is part one of my twenty-eight-day fasting program. If you have psoriasis, you probably have significantly increased intestinal permeability as well as an increased toxic burden on your liver. It is critically important to repair your GI tract and detoxify your liver, which a rice protein fast helps to accomplish. It is also extremely important to avoid foods to which you are allergic.

Patients with eczema are usually sensitive to dairy and peanuts, so these foods need to be eliminated. Patients with psoriasis are many times sensitive to nightshades (tomatoes, potatoes, peppers, and eggplant), red meat, pork, shellfish, dairy, and fried food. Therefore these foods should be eliminated.

HYPERTENSION

Do you have high blood pressure? One of the best ways to treat hypertension is to go on a juice fast. Before your fast, you should first attempt to get off all medications under medical supervision. Increase the amount of clean, pure water (not tap water) you drink to at least two to three quarts a day. Follow the directions for the detoxification fast outlined in this book and the instructions in my book *The Bible Cure for High Blood Pressure*.[2]

FOR COLDS AND FLU

When you come down with a cold or flu, fast by drinking plenty of water and fresh juices, and get plenty of rest. This will help your system to expel toxic materials through the mucus it creates. Let your fever burn up your infection, too. Don't rush to the doctor and take a lot of medications to halt the symptoms. Some of them are important for detoxification. However, if you have a fever over 102 degrees, you should be examined by a physician. If your fever is greater than 101 degrees and persists for longer than a few days, you should also be examined by a physician. For children, seek medical attention sooner.

You can overcome many infectious diseases by eliminating all dairy products. Also eliminate mucus-forming foods such as eggs and processed grains. These grains include pancakes, cereals, doughnuts, white bread, crackers, pretzels, bagels, white rice, gravies, cakes, and pies. In addition, cut out consumption of margarine, butter, and other saturated, hydrogenated, and processed oils. Also avoid sweets such as candies, cookies, cakes, pies, doughnuts, and so forth.

When you are sick, don't instantly turn to antibiotics. Antibiotics can provide powerful help when you are very ill with a bacterial infection. But the overuse of antibiotics can harm you and has created resistant strains of bacteria. Realize that antibiotics will not treat viruses, which cause the vast majority of infections.

Many doctors prescribe antibiotics for colds and flus that do not even respond to antibiotics. If you have had a fever as described earlier, go see your doctor. But don't insist on getting an antibiotic unless he or she strongly recommends it. For more information, refer to *The Bible Cure for Colds, Flu and Sinus Infections.*[3]

Let your body's own immune system be your first defense against infections. Overusing antibiotics creates yeast and bad bacteria overgrowth in the intestinal tract, an increased risk of developing impaired intestinal permeability, and an increased toxic burden on the liver.

These are some of the amazing physical results you can experience through regular fasting. But this discussion on fasting and detoxification would be incomplete if we left out the most important aspect of fasting and purification—fasting for the soul and spirit. For you see, the work of fasting doesn't stop with the physical body—fasting cleanses the total person. Let's take a look at fasting's greatest, most powerful work: cleansing the soul.

CHAPTER 6

Recognizing the Spiritual Power of Regular Fasting

Fasting is more than just a powerful method for cleansing and healing your physical body. It is also a tool for cleansing the soul. Fasting is a key to genuine and deep spirituality. Throughout the ages, people have used fasting as a tool for entering into deeper spiritual realms and getting to know God better. In the Bible, fasting was considered a key part of entering into and maintaining a powerful and spiritually dynamic walk with God.

To fast biblically, you must voluntarily abstain from food—partially or completely—for a period of time *for a spiritual purpose.* During a spiritual fast, you deny yourself one of the most basic elements of survival, one that is loved and cherished by your body—food.

Just why would any one of us even want to consider denying our body the cookies, cakes, ice cream, hamburgers, and pizza it so much enjoys? The reason is that fasting, when accomplished through the direction and enabling of the Holy Spirit, has the power to break the gripping control of our lower nature.

UNDERSTANDING OUR TRUE NATURE

Our fleshly appetite can be a ravenous animal, overpowering the spiritual man within us. When this happens, it seems impossible to say no to a craving for sweets, fast food—or even sex, gossip, or slander. These strong cravings and desires are a part of our lower, baser, or more animal-like nature. The Bible uses the term *flesh* when it speaks about these cravings and desires of our bodies, and it warns us that we must conquer these appetites. These desires include the following:

- Laziness and lethargy that keeps us from exercising

- Cravings for sweets and fats that cause us to eat too much of all the wrong foods so that we end up piling on the extra pounds and never properly nourishing our bodies

- Out-of-control emotions such as anger and rage that can send us into a frenzy in traffic or cause us to say hurtful things to our loved ones, which we later regret

- Loneliness, anxiety, depression, and grief that may trigger us to seek comfort in sugary, starchy foods

Many more things come under the category of flesh. It can involve our thoughts, our emotions, our desires for inappropriate sex, our compulsion to binge out on sweets, our inability to stop ourselves from gossiping, and much, much more. Flesh is nothing more than our needs, wants, and cravings in their undisciplined state.

FASTING CONTROLS THE LOWER NATURE

Since we are all born with these undisciplined needs, wants, and cravings, the key to our spirituality is yielding to the Spirit of God. The Bible encourages us to walk in the presence and power of the Spirit as an anecdote for living in the flesh. In Galatians 5:16–17, Paul says:

I say then: Walk in the Spirit, and you shall not fulfill the lust of the flesh. For the flesh lusts against the Spirit, and the Spirit against the flesh; and these are contrary to one another, so that you do not do the things that you wish.

The carnal, unrenewed mind of the flesh is controlled and dominated by the thinking and reasoning of our intellects. Emotions also control and dominate this lower nature, which means that your feelings and desires control you. In addition to that, the carnal nature is also controlled by the five senses of taste, smell, sight, feeling, and hearing.

But there is hope. The power of God is released through the Holy Spirit who works in us. Ephesians 3:20 tells us, "Now to Him who is able to do exceedingly abundantly above all that we ask or think, according to the power that works in us..." It's only as we live our lives in vital connection with God that we become able to crucify the lusts of the flesh and live and walk in the higher nature of the Spirit of God within.

This process of crucifying the flesh must be accomplished daily through prayer, forgiving anyone who wrongs us (including ourselves), renewing the mind by regularly reading the Word of God, and by watching every word that comes out of our mouths. All of these things are like the hammers, pickaxes, drills, and machinery that operate at the rock quarry of our hardened flesh. In this effort, fasting is the dynamite that makes all of the other efforts easier and more effective.

When the bathroom scale tells us that we need to lose weight, but we find it woefully impossible not to reach for one more slice of chocolate cake or bowl of ice cream, then we are encountering this powerful grip of our flesh. It has gained prominence over our mind, will, spirit, and emotions.

One way to break the power of your flesh and bring it under submission to your spirit and mind is to fast. Do you have an out-of-control temper that flares up at all the worst moments, damaging relationships with those you love? Fasting can bring that flesh under control.

Fasting feeds your spirit man while starving your natural man. It can soften your heart and cleanse your body to make you more receptive to God's plans. Fasting can sensitize your spirit to discern the voice and internal promptings of God's Spirit. Let's take a look at some more spiritual applications of fasting.

WHY WE SHOULD FAST SPIRITUALLY

Fasting builds godly character

For starters, fasting builds character. By enabling us to surrender our lives to God in greater measure, we find more control over our tongues, our minds, our attitudes, our emotions, our bodies, and all our fleshly desires. Fasting also helps us to submit our spirits to God completely so that He can use them for His purposes.

Even though many Christians have invited the power of the Holy Spirit into their lives, they continue to be led about by the insatiable appetites of the flesh. They live their lives pursuing whatever gratifies the cravings of the lower nature or their own selfish motives instead of the purposes of God. Many are good people who actually would like to live on a much higher plane of existence, but they just don't know how.

Fasting gives us the ability to build up character and integrity by allowing the Spirit of God to operate through us. The only real way to build godly character and genuine integrity into our inner man is by spending time in the presence of God.

Fasting loosens the chains of bondage

Do you struggle with addictions or addictive behaviors? Sometimes addictions can even show up in our personalities rather than through debilitating behaviors such as alcoholism. For instance, perhaps you have never been an alcoholic, but when you get into a room filled with people, you have an obsessive need to be constantly talking or running everything and everyone in sight. An exaggerated need to control others or to control circumstances and situations can be just as much of a bondage as a drug addiction.

Bondage comes in all shapes, colors, types, and sizes. So don't be too quick to dismiss the notion that you may have some type of bondage in your own life. Most of us growing up and living in this imperfect world end up with some type of bondage—or we know someone struggling to be free from destructive, addictive behaviors. Perhaps you can think of loved ones who are bound by addictive personalities or behaviors. Fasting is critically important if you have children who need to be set free from drugs and alcohol, homosexuality, pornography, or some form of rebellion. Fasting can be extremely helpful when you are praying for a loved one's salvation. Fasting can begin to break any spiritual stronghold so that peace and harmony can return.

Fasting humbles us

Although the lower nature can seem amazingly powerful, fasting humbles it. Humbling the flesh is required if we want to live a clean, godly life.

> Therefore whoever humbles himself as this little child is the greatest in the kingdom of heaven.
> —MATTHEW 18:4

> Therefore humble yourselves under the mighty hand of God, that He may exalt you in due time.
> —1 PETER 5:6

> Humble yourselves in the sight of the Lord, and He will lift you up.
> —JAMES 4:10

And whoever exalts himself will be humbled, and he who humbles himself will be exalted.

—MATTHEW 23:12

Fasting gets God's attention because it is a key to humility. When we humble our flesh, we find favor with God. James 4:6 says, "God resists the proud, but gives grace to the humble." In other words, the humility that can be obtained through spiritual fasting opens the door to God's grace and favor.

Fasting helps us enter the presence of God

Have you ever desired to experience God's presence? Fasting can bring the healing and refreshing presence of God into an individual life and into the life of a family or even a nation.

After Moses fasted for forty days, he was swept up into an entirely new place in God's Spirit. He received the Ten Commandments and became the lawgiver of Israel. After Jesus had fasted for forty days, the Holy Spirit empowered His life, and His ministry of healing and preaching was launched.

You too can receive the touch of God's glory upon your own life, just as Jesus and Moses did, through fasting and prayer. Fasting enables us to touch the world around us with God's love and power. Fasting can be a tool to access God's power to affect our children, our extended families, our cities, and even the world.

Fasting brings divine guidance

When you are making critical decisions such as choosing your mate, changing a job, deciding to move, or other major life-impacting decisions, you need God's divine guidance to be sure you are not holding onto opinions or other judgments that are in error. The problem with error is that when we are in it, we think we are right. That's why we need divine guidance for life's major decisions.

The Bible promises that the Holy Spirit is ready and willing to provide that guidance when you ask.

> However, when He, the Spirit of truth, has come, He will guide you into all truth; for He will not speak on His own authority, but whatever He hears He will speak; and He will tell you things to come.
>
> —JOHN 16:13

There are times in all of our lives when we are being led around by our own misjudgments and desires, and we don't even know it. Regular fasting can protect us from the blindness of our own opinions and desires.

Fasting will help us to be led by the Spirit instead of being led by faulty judgments. That's why spiritual fasting is so very important.

Fasting brings healing

Fasting is also a powerful tool for healing and restoration. Here is what the Bible says about it:

> Then your light shall break forth like the morning, your healing shall spring forth speedily, and your righteousness shall go before you; the glory of the Lord shall be your rear guard.
>
> —ISAIAH 58:8

Not only does fasting break the chains of wickedness, lift heavy burdens, and free the oppressed, but it also brings back your health.

WHEN WE SHOULD FAST SPIRITUALLY

Always fast as the Holy Spirit leads. In other words, just as Jesus was led into the wilderness to fast and pray, we should also be led by the Spirit into times and seasons of fasting. The New Testament never lays down strict rules regarding fasting; therefore, we should never impose strict rules upon others or ourselves. Legalistic fasting earned the Pharisee in the Book of Luke no brownie points with God. The times and reasons for our spiritual fasting are to be directed by God and not man.

God is most concerned with our motives for fasting. Jesus too was far more concerned with the motives behind fasting than with how long or how often we fast. Motive is everything when it comes to spiritual fasting.

As you develop a life of fasting and prayer, you will find that God will lead and guide you. You will walk in the footsteps of great men and women who have gone before us—men and women who increased in purity of body, mind, and spirit and who touched heaven with their prayers and nations with their passions. Daniel was one of these men. His fasting brought about powerful results. Let's take a look at the Daniel fast for overcoming the flesh.

FOLLOW DANIEL'S EXAMPLE

A Daniel fast is a partial fast based on the way Daniel and three other Hebrew youths fasted when the Jews were taken captive and led away to Babylon. Daniel and his three friends were greatly favored for their purity, and they were well educated and extremely gifted both mentally and spiritually.

When these four young men were taken into the king's palace to be educated in the ways of the Chaldeans, Daniel 1:5 states, "The king assigned them a daily amount of food and wine from the king's table" (NIV). He planned to keep them on his own rich diet of meats, fats, sugary pastries, and wine for three years. At the end of the three years, they would be presented to the king.

However, verse 8 says, "But Daniel resolved not to defile himself with the royal food and wine" (NIV). In other words, Daniel rejected the rich, tempting delicious meats, wine, and pastries of the royal court, perhaps because they did not meet the requirements of Jewish dietary laws or because these youths may have taken vows against drinking alcohol.

So Daniel made a request of the prince of the eunuchs. Verses 11–12 say, "Daniel then said… 'Please test your servants for ten days: Give us nothing but vegetables to eat and water to drink'" (NIV). The King James Version uses the word *pulse* to describe what Daniel and his friends ate. Strong's concordance defines *pulse* as "vegetables eaten as food." I believe the Daniel fast was all vegetables and no grains, meat, or wine. Peas, beans, and lentils are also known as pulses. Pulses are high in protein, carbohydrates, and fiber. They are also low in fat, which is mainly unsaturated fat.

The twenty-eight-day fast in this book incorporates what I call a modified Daniel fast. We have eliminated everything that Daniel eliminated except some of the non-gluten whole grains. If you desire to modify this fast to a true Daniel fast, I recommend that you stick to the salad and soup recipes I've provided, being sure to eliminate any and all grain products. You can also enjoy the recipes provided for the week of juice fasting while observing a Daniel fast.

Daniel and the three Hebrew young men lived a fasted life for three years on the vegetarian diet of pulse while learning and studying in the king's court, and God honored their partial fast. We're told in verse 15, "At the end of the ten days they looked healthier and better nourished than any of the young men who ate the royal food" (NIV).

God tremendously favored their decision to fast and granted them favor, wisdom, and insight far above anyone around them. In verses 18–20 (NIV) we read:

> At the end of the time set by the king to bring them in, the chief official presented them to Nebuchadnezzar. The king talked with them, and he found none equal to Daniel, Hananiah, Mishael, and Azariah; so they entered the king's service. In every matter of wisdom and understanding about which the king questioned them, he found them ten times better than all the magicians and enchanters in his whole kingdom.

Daniel knew what was healthy to eat, and he purposed in his heart that he would not defile himself. The Daniel fast eliminates rich foods that are tempting to the flesh.

Today, people are so bound to their flesh that they often cannot go one meal without eating some form of meat, something sweet, something fatty, or some other type of rich food. We must crucify our flesh daily and take up our cross and follow Christ. (See Matthew 16:24.) What better way to crucify our flesh than to follow Daniel's fasted lifestyle?

I recommend that you follow the complete twenty-eight-day fasting program for detoxification as outlined for you in the next section. But as you set out on a lifestyle of regular fasting, you may, at times, want to adapt the first twenty-one days of this detoxification fast to conform to the guidelines of a Daniel fast. To do so, simply stick to the recipes for salads, soups, and juices provided in this book and be sure to eliminate any and all grain products (millet, barley, spelt, quinoa, oats, etc.).

PREPARE YOURSELF FOR SPIRITUAL GROWTH

Fasting is a privilege, and it is a biblical key to cleansing that will bless your life. The Bible gives fasting an ancient position of honor, a place beside other dynamic principles for health and spiritual growth. As you undergo this time of fasting, prayer, personal reflection, and spiritual growth, here are some considerations that will help you to prepare your heart.

- First, commit the time of your fast to God for spiritual cleansing and renewal.

- Next, set aside a portion of each day to read the Bible, meditate on what you read, and ask the Holy Spirit, your Teacher, to give you divine revelation.

- As your body becomes accustomed to the fast, consider devoting increased portions of your time to Bible reading, prayer, and journaling for personal and spiritual growth.

- Listen to Bible teaching tapes while you're driving, at work, or at home to help you stay focused on God's Word.

- Pray as often as possible, or do as Scripture says and pray without ceasing.

- There may also be times when you choose to commit your fast to a higher purpose, such as fasting for issues of national cleansing and healing.

YOUR FASTING JOURNAL

The third section of this book will walk you through the twenty-eight days of my detoxification fasting program. Chapter seven includes a daily plan for the twenty-one-day partial fast that will support your liver in cleansing and detoxifying your body, and chapter eight includes a daily plan for the seven-day juice fast. The pages of the fasting program have been designed to imitate a daily journal that incorporates several things that will help you grow and develop as a total person—body, mind, and spirit—as you learn to fast.

Each day of the journal will provide you with dietary guidelines and encouragement for the physical aspects of your fast, but it will also focus on a different spiritual benefit of fasting found in the Bible. Each journal entry also includes a place for you to record your prayers, prayer requests, thoughts, and insights. Here are some pointers that will also help:

- Take time to be quiet before the Lord, and listen to the voice of the Spirit.

- Record in your journal what the Holy Spirit is revealing to you.

- Write down revelation and insights given to you during the fast.

- Write down praise reports.

- Write down any dreams, and pray for the interpretation of them.

As you set aside time for reflecting, journaling, prayer, and Bible reading during your fast period, you will begin to touch the dynamic benefits of fasting for the cleansing and healing of the heart, mind, body, and spirit. Now, let's turn the page and begin our program.

GET
HEALTHY

CHAPTER 7

Supporting My Liver With Nutrition

This chapter is an introduction to the first part of my twenty-eight-day fasting program. It will provide you with the information you need to prepare for the actual fasting part of this detoxification and cleansing program. Before you consider fasting, it is important to follow this uniquely designed nutritional program to strengthen and support your liver, which will prepare it for the increased role of detoxification during your fast.

Your body was uniquely created to handle enormous amounts of toxins, poisons, germs, and diseases. Your body's detoxification system, including your liver and GI tract, is astonishingly powerful. With proper nutritional support from you, it is able to both detoxify and eliminate chemicals and toxins.

The benefits to you of a detoxification system that is functioning at peak efficiency are unending. A properly operating detoxification system in your body will:

- Prevent and even reverse disease

- Provide you with more energy

- Allow you to feel better

- Aid you in losing weight

- Help clear up your skin and complexion

The first system of toxic cleansing is your liver. It's an amazing organ that works day and night to cleanse your blood from chemicals, poisons, bacteria, virus, and any other foreign invader that comes to rob you of your good health. If your liver is not strong and healthy, you will not be strong and healthy. That's why it is so important for you to spend the first twenty-one days of my fasting program strengthening your liver so it can carry out its key role in the detoxification process.

If you wanted to be an Olympic award-winning athlete, you wouldn't enter the competition without spending months in training, strengthening your muscles, developing your skills, and building your body with the best diet and nutrition available. Well, in the same way, you must train your body to compete against the toxic world in which you live. The good news is that it's a competition you can win. But you have an enormous part in ensuring the long-term successful outcome.

FACTOID:

Certain foods increase the capacity of the liver to detoxify our bodies of harmful substances—foods such as wasabi (the green, spicy paste served with sushi), broccoli, cabbage, brussels sprouts, kale, and cauliflower.

YOUR TWENTY-ONE-DAY LIVER SUPPORT PROGRAM

For the first three weeks of my fasting program, you will follow this diet and regimen of supplements to prepare your body for fasting. It would even be very beneficial for you to restore your body following the fasting part of the program by repeating another one-week liver support diet.

These dietary guidelines will help cleanse and support your liver while you fast and will continue helping your body to operate at peak efficiency as you begin your health-first lifestyle at the conclusion of my fasting program. The more closely you follow these guidelines, the more benefit you will receive from your fast. It is important that you change your diet and lifestyle to reduce the amount of toxins you are taking in as well as improve your body's ability to eliminate toxins.

This first twenty-one days of my fasting program will give you the necessary dietary guidelines to cleanse and support your liver before your begin the juice fast part of the program. To get the optimum benefit, be careful to strictly follow these guidelines.

FOODS TO AVOID

Making the right choices of food for your liver's health is important, especially before you consider detoxification through fasting. Here are some foods (and other products) to avoid:

- Colas and chocolate

- Alcohol (including wine)

- Processed vegetable oils

- Animal skins and meats

- Deep-fried foods

- Microwaved foods

- Hydrogenated and partially hydrogenated fats and oils, which are always found in most commercial peanut butter, margarine, and shortening but are also often included in foods such as bread, cake mixes, frozen foods, breakfast cereals, potato chips, and more (read all labels carefully)

- Refined foods and processed foods, including white bread, chips, cereals, instant oatmeal, and instant rice

- Simple sugars, including honey, pastries, cookies, candies, cakes, and pies

- Fast foods

- Processed juices

- Wheat products, including crackers, bagels, pasta, muffins (sprouted breads such as Ezekiel or manna bread are OK)

- Corn products

- Soy products

- Dairy products, including butter, cheese, milk, yogurt, sour cream, and ice cream

- Eggs

- Fish and poultry

- Individuals with autoimmune diseases such as psoriasis, rheumatoid arthritis, and lupus may need to avoid nightshades (tomatoes, potatoes, eggplant, and peppers), since these foods may aggravate their condition.

For this detoxification fasting program, I have eliminated all meat, dairy, eggs, and other foods that commonly trigger allergic reactions or food sensitivity reactions, including corn, soy, wheat, and processed foods. Sprouted breads such as Ezekiel and manna bread are allowed unless you are sensitive to gluten, which is the protein in wheat.

FOODS TO EAT

For at least two weeks, in preparation for your fast, eat as many of the following foods as possible. Because certain fruits and vegetables have higher pesticide residues than others, and I strongly recommend organic for these.

- Organic fruit: Drink a glass of freshly juiced fruits and vegetables in the morning.

- Organic vegetables: Eat as many raw vegetables as possible. In addition, cruciferous vegetables, such as cabbage, cauliflower, brussels sprouts, broccoli, kale, collard greens, mustard greens, and turnips, are very important. Other liver-friendly vegetables include legumes (all types of beans), beets, carrots, dandelion root, and greens. You may steam the veggies or lightly stir-fry them in organic extra-virgin coconut, macadamia nut, or olive oil.

- Liver-friendly starches: Eat brown rice, wild rice, rice pasta, and brown rice bread.

- Good fats for your liver and for detoxification: Use organic, extra-virgin olive oil; avocados; raw, fresh nuts such as almonds, macadamia nuts, and walnuts (avoid peanuts and cashews); seeds; flaxseed oil (not for cooking); evening primrose oil; black currant seed oil; borage oil; and fish oil.

- Beverages: Drink plenty of pure, clean water with fresh-squeezed lemon or lime (two quarts daily), fresh vegetable and fruit juices, organic green tea or black tea, and other herbal teas. While I don't recommend that you start drinking organic coffee, one cup of organic coffee per day is allowable if you are already a coffee drinker when you begin the program.

SUPPLEMENTS FOR THE LIVER

There are certain supplements that are very important to the liver, which you should take to prepare for a detoxification fast and when ending a fast. For a complete discussion of important liver supplements, please see my book *Toxic Relief.* Following is a summary of the important supplements that I recommend you take every day of the first twenty-one days—the liver support phase—of this fasting program. (See Appendix B for a list of brand names for each supplement.)

- A comprehensive multivitamin and mineral supplement

- Milk thistle (Silybin Phytosome)

- NAC (N-acetyl cysteine)

- Organic green tea, dandelion tea, other herb teas (available at health food stores)

- Phytonutrient powder/drink

- Balanced rice protein supplement (optional): one scoop in 4 ounces of water, twice a day, for those individuals who are sensitive to fruits or vegetables or who have a sensitive GI tract

IT TAKES A POSITIVE ATTITUDE

The successful completion of this fasting program requires a winning attitude and the support of your friends and loved ones! Not only do you need a determined attitude to make necessary lifestyle changes, but also it will be very important to maintain a positive and cheerful outlook as well.

Discuss this part of the fasting program with your family. Whether or not they are joining you in this twenty-eight-day program, it is best to discuss the program with them first. This would be an excellent time to sit down together as a family and create the guidelines for your new health-first lifestyle that you will launch at the end of the twenty-eight days. A supportive family and supportive friends working together and encouraging each other throughout the fasting program and on into your new lifestyle are a powerful force for success.

As you begin this phase, it is extremely important now for you to make the decision to eliminate toxins from your life. This should be a permanent decision for you, and it is essential during the twenty-eight-day fasting program. Avoid cigarette smoke, alcohol, and drugs. Decrease your intake of all medications. Of course, for prescription medicines, you must do this with your doctor's help. Be sensible; never make drastic changes without consulting your doctor.

OTHER TIPS AND TECHNIQUES

- Do not cut or prepare fruits and vegetables before you are ready to eat them. You may be tempted to slice up that melon and carrot just for the convenience of being able to grab them from the refrigerator, but fruits and vegetables lose their nutrients when they are cut and stored. It's best to prepare them when you know they will be immediately eaten.

- Don't deplete your food of nutrients by improper cooking techniques. When you boil vegetables, most of the nutrients leave the vegetables and end up in the water. By the time you eat them, the boiled water has a greater nutrient content than the vegetables themselves! (Soups, however, are an exception to this rule because you do consume the broth that contains the nutrients from the vegetables.)

- If you must boil vegetables, bring the water to a boil first and then add your veggies to the water for a brief time. Do not allow them to soak in the water. Drain them immediately and serve them. I strongly recommend steaming your vegetables or eating them raw. I also recommend that my patients avoid microwaved foods altogether.

- Don't prepare too much food or prepare it too far ahead of time. Reheating food and leftovers depletes the food of valuable vitamins, minerals, and other nutrients—especially if you reheat in the microwave. A study in *Science News* in 1998 found that just six minutes of microwave cooking destroyed half the vitamin B_{12} in dairy foods and meat, a much higher rate of destruction than other cooking techniques.[1]

- Fruits and vegetables should be eaten unpeeled whenever possible because many vitamins and minerals are actually concentrated just beneath their skin. If you have not purchased organic items, it is imperative that you wash these fruits and vegetables carefully to remove pesticides. (See chapter eight for information on washing fruits and vegetables.)

- It is best to use fresh, organically grown produce. However, if fresh products are not available, choose frozen fruits and vegetables. Only rarely should you choose canned fruits and vegetables, making sure the label lists only organic, whole ingredients.

> **FACTOID:**
> Your mother may have taught you that the best vitamins are found in the skin of the potato—but so are the pesticides. Don't eat the potato skins unless you use organically grown potatoes.

- I have found that many of my patients benefit from a supplement called Beano after eating beans, lentils, peas, or cruciferous vegetables (broccoli, cabbage, cauliflower, and brussels sprouts). It is simply an enzyme that enables you to digest beans and certain vegetables.

BEFORE YOU BEGIN

Before you start, it's important to set the boundaries of your fast. Determine what type of fast you will go on. Check the boxes below that identify fast or fasts you will be implementing.

☐ A partial fast to support the liver during detoxification

☐ A Daniel fast, as in the book of Daniel (See chapter six for more information on substituting the liver support fast with a Daniel fast.)

☐ A fruit and vegetable juice fast

One final note: As you look through the daily meal plans, keep in mind that these are only suggestions provided to give you variety. All of the recipes are provided in the back of this book and are grouped by meal type. This will allow you to substitute and/or repeat any meal within a given meal type (breakfast, lunch, dinner, snack) according to your tastes. I do ask that you limit yourself to the recipes given in this book and that you follow the recipes exactly as written in order to ensure that you receive the benefits of detoxifying your body.

I would like to thank Ed and Elisa McClure, founders of the ZOE 8 Weight Management Program and authors of *Eat Your Way to a Healthy Life*,[2] for contributing many of the recipes for our fasting program. Any recipe title followed by an asterisk (*) indicates that it is a ZOE 8 recipe.

Now it's time to get started. I pray that these special days of cleansing and healing will be some of the most rewarding days of your entire life. I pray that you will experience renewed health, energy, and vitality. In addition, I pray that your soul and spirit will be refreshed and renewed.

CLEANSING AND DETOX FAST
Days 1–21

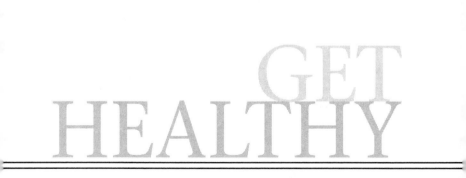

GET
HEALTHY

DAY 1

DR. COLBERT'S CLEANSING AND DETOX FAST

MEAL SUGGESTIONS

Breakfast	Snack	Lunch	Dinner
Easy Breakfast Wraps (page 143)	Spicy Sunflower Seeds (page 151)	Cucumber-Sprout Salad (page 159)	Vegetarian Chili* (page 169)

FOCUS THOUGHT

Without a healthy, well-functioning liver and a healthy intestinal tract, your body will continue to labor under a dangerous burden of toxins.

YOUR DAILY PRESCRIPTION FOR HEALTH

With a special diet to get your liver and GI tract in shape, and a program of short, easy juice fasts, together with some lifestyle changes, you really can cleanse your body. By cleansing your system of built-up toxins, you truly will feel better than you have in years. Deep cleansing your body right down to the cellular level will renew your vitality, restore your energy, reclaim your health, shed toxic fat, lengthen your life, and give you a healthy glow.

YOUR DAILY SPIRITUAL JOURNEY

And those who are Christ's have crucified the flesh with its passions and desires. If we live in the Spirit, let us also walk in the Spirit.

—GALATIANS 5:24–25

Fasting is a powerful spiritual tool that helps us to see with spiritual eyes. It clears our vision and helps us to focus on the things of God. He has so many things to give us, but sometimes we miss out because we put our attention elsewhere. Allow Him to redirect your thoughts and desires and align them with His purposes today. As you begin this period of self-denial, I encourage you to read Galatians 5:16–26 as a refresher of what it means to walk in the Spirit and do war with your flesh—every part of you that is affected by sin.

Think about the physical and spiritual reasons for your fast, and write a statement about why you are beginning this twenty-eight-day fasting program and what you hope will be accomplished during this special time.

_____

_____

_____

Now that you have thought about your purpose(s) for fasting, it is time to make a commitment to stick with the program. Here's a prayer of declaration. To help you stay committed, I encourage you to say this prayer (or a similar one in your own words) aloud with conviction before every meal during your fast.

Dear Lord, no longer will I only use my willpower to control my eating; instead I will use Your power infused into my willpower through the Holy Spirit. I will crucify my flesh daily and give my body what it needs and not what it craves. From this day on, I refuse to pollute my body by eating unhealthy food. I boldly confess that, with the Holy Spirit's help, I will cleanse and detoxify my body, His temple. In Jesus' name, amen.

RECORD YOUR THOUGHTS

Use the space below to record what you sense God is laying on your heart about this time of fasting or any prayer requests that you are bringing to Him during this time.

_____

_____

_____

DAY 2

DR. COLBERT'S CLEANSING AND DETOX FAST

MEAL SUGGESTIONS

Breakfast	Snack	Lunch	Dinner
Cinnamon Oats (page 144)	Granola Crumble (page 151)	Tomato-Bean Salad with Garlic Bread* (pages 159, 183)	Quinoa Tabouli* and Roasted Bell Peppers* (page 170)

FOCUS THOUGHT

It is important to understand that your thinking patterns and emotional responses affect your body. God desires for you to be totally well, physically, mentally, emotionally, and spiritually.

YOUR DAILY PRESCRIPTION FOR HEALTH

Fasting provides your body, mind, and spirit with many benefits. Medical science is recognizing more and more the innate connection between these inseparable facets of our being. What we eat affects our moods and, to a certain extent, even our attitudes. What we think affects how our bodies digest food and impacts the way we handle stress. And our spiritual well-being is influenced by our physical and mental health. Toxic emotions such as anger, resentment, fear, anxiety, grief, and depression can create excessive stress, whereas positive emotions such as gratitude, joy, love, and peace actually relieve stress. The physical effects of reprogramming your thoughts begin with your heart. Your heartbeat varies from moment to moment, based on your emotions and attitudes. When you experience stress and negative emotions such as anger, frustration, fear, and anxiety, your heart rate variability pattern becomes more erratic and disordered, and it sends chaotic signals to the brain. The result is energy drain and added wear and tear on your mind and body. In contrast, sustained positive emotions such as appreciateion, love, joy, and compassion are associated with highly ordered heart rate patterns and a significant reduction of stress.

YOUR DAILY SPIRITUAL JOURNEY

Keep your heart with all diligence, for out of it spring the issues of life.
—PROVERBS 4:23

Dedicate this time of fasting to focus yourself on the things God has done in your life. In the space provided, make a list of things for which you are thankful. Include your physical well-being—your eyesight, your hearing, and your ability to taste, smell, and touch. Be grateful you have the use of your fingers, hands, arms, legs, and so on. Don't forget to thank Him for modern-day conveniences such as a car, running hot water, air conditioning and heat, a working computer, telephone, and more. Thank God for meeting your everyday needs—food, water, clothing, transportation, and shelter. Thank Him for loved ones to care about, such as your spouse, children, relatives, friends, co-workers—even your pets! Finally, thank Him for nature—flowers, weather, fresh air, anything that makes you grateful to be alive.

_____

_____

_____

Review this list daily, update it as needed, and recite it aloud. You can also pray this prayer (or something similar in your own words).

Dear Lord, I ask You to help me to keep my heart free from wrong attitudes and emotions. Instead of complaining about things that I don't have, I choose to be grateful for the many blessings that I do have. I choose today to let go of negative thoughts and lies from the enemy of my soul. Help me to stand on the promises in Your Word and think on things that are based on Your truth. In Jesus' name, amen.

RECORD YOUR THOUGHTS

Use the space below to record the thoughts that have come to your mind during today's prayer time.

_____

_____

_____

_____

MEAL SUGGESTIONS

Breakfast	Snack	Lunch	Dinner
Muesli* (page 144)	Spicy Chickpeas (page 152)	Un-Caesar Salad (page 160)	Broccoli Italian Style,* Dill Potatoes, and Black Bean Burgers (page 171)

FOCUS THOUGHT

Forgiveness enables the body to release toxins. Choose to extend forgiveness today—this includes forgiving yourself.

YOUR DAILY PRESCRIPTION FOR HEALTH

Many individuals rehash, relive, and meditate on painful experiences of their past. They relive the hurt over and over, and they never heal. These individuals are harboring an offense—a circumstance that is perceived as unjust or hurtful. When you harbor an offense, you usually deal with the problem by thinking about it too much and talking about it too much. The sad thing is that holding unforgiveness in your heart literally locks toxins inside your body. When you fail to forgive, you stimulate the stress response in your body. This causes chronic stimulation of the sympathetic nervous system and elevation of stress hormones, which in turn causes constriction of blood vessels and locks toxins in the body. For more information on this topic please refer to my book *Deadly Emotions*.[3]

YOUR DAILY SPIRITUAL JOURNEY

You must make allowance for each other's faults and forgive the person who offends you. Remember, the Lord forgave you, so you must forgive others.
—COLOSSIANS 3:13, NLT

One of the great spiritual benefits of fasting is that it can bring reconciliation and restoration into our lives. Let this be your focus today. As you spend time in prayer, the Holy Spirit may prompt you to seek reconciliation and restoration from someone who has wronged you. Ask God to show you any person or people to whom you must go and seek reconciliation. What are their names?

_____

_____

_____

Forgiving is simply letting go of old hurts and releasing people and situations into God's hands. It is helpful to first picture the person whom you need to forgive with your eyes closed; then when you can see his or her face, forgive him or her by praying the following prayer below (or a similar one in your own words).

Father, I acknowledge that I have sinned against You by not forgiving those who have offended me. Lord, You forgave me and canceled my debt; therefore, I can forgive anyone who has hurt me. I also acknowledge my inability to forgive them apart from You. Therefore, with Your help and from my heart, I choose to forgive [[fill in the name]]. I cancel their debt; they no longer owe me anything. I ask that You bless them and lead them into a closer relationship with You. In Jesus' name, amen.

In the same way, forgive others, one by one, including yourself, God, parents, in-laws, grandparents, siblings, spouse, ex-spouse(s), children, and any others who have offended you, whether you remember specific events related to each one or not.

RECORD YOUR THOUGHTS

Use the space below to write anything you've discovered about forgiveness today.

_____

_____

_____

_____

MEAL SUGGESTIONS

Breakfast	Snack	Lunch	Dinner
Tex-Mex Bagels (page 144)	Brown rice crackers and Asparagus Tapenade* (page 152)	Quinoa Crunch Salad (page 160)	Gazpacho* and Garlic Bread* (pages 170, 183)

FOCUS THOUGHT

Let what you take into your body provide healing. "Let your medicine be your food, and let your food be your medicine" (Hippocrates).

YOUR DAILY PRESCRIPTION FOR HEALTH

Fasting is good for you on so many levels. There are few things you can do for your body that have as much power to radically improve your physical health as fasting has. Fasting helps to break food addictions and other unhealthy eating habits. After a fast, fresh fruits and vegetables taste wonderful. And you won't desire to "binge" or overeat as you receive the nourishment your body needs. So don't be alarmed. Fasting doesn't have to be scary. It will improve your health physically and spiritually.

YOUR DAILY SPIRITUAL JOURNEY

Your healing shall spring forth speedily.

—ISAIAH 58:8

There is great spiritual power in fasting. It enables you to be released from things that have been keeping you from all God has for you. One of these things is sickness. You may fast to bring healing to your own body, or you may fast for the illness of loved one. List the physical burdens and people for whom you are fasting.

_____

_____

_____

Now it's time to pray for healing, speaking words of life. I like to call it "praying the answer, not the problem." Instead of identifying yourself with certain illnesses and diseases ("Lord, please heal 'my' arthritis," "Lord, heal 'my' diabetes," etc.), pray the answer as promised in God's Word. Here's an example of what I mean.

Father, in Isaiah 53:5, Your Word promises that because of Jesus' stripes, I am healed. As I focus on the amazing love of Christ who suffered and died for me, help me to remember that in addition to my salvation, He also purchased my healing. I am healed. I receive the promise of healing in Jesus by faith. Amen.

Pray this prayer, or use your own words. Spend a few moments in silence, meditating on the promises of healing God has given in His Word.

RECORD YOUR THOUGHTS

Use the space below to record what you sense the Holy Spirit is laying on your heart—perhaps through thoughts or images in your mind—during this quiet time.

_____

_____

_____

MEAL SUGGESTIONS

Breakfast	Snack	Lunch	Dinner
Buckwheat Pancakes (page 145)	Cajun Nut Mix* (page 152)	Garbanzo Bean Salad* (page 161)	Rice Pasta With Lentil Sauce and Garlic Bread* (pages 172, 183)

FOCUS THOUGHT

You can wean yourself from unhealthy eating habits by consciously substituting "dead" food products that have been old favorites of yours with "living foods." For example, choose Ezekiel or manna bread instead of white bread.

YOUR DAILY PRESCRIPTION FOR HEALTH

"Living foods"—organic fruits, vegetables, whole grains, nuts, and seeds—produce life. Man-made food is generally "dead," meaning it has no enzymes and will usually be deficient in vitamins, minerals, antioxidants, and phytonutrients. "Dead foods" include most fast foods, sugary foods, processed foods, junk foods, and snack foods. Excessive intake of dead foods eventually leads to degenerative diseases and early death.

YOUR DAILY SPIRITUAL JOURNEY

You shall be called the Repairer of the Breach, the Restorer of Streets to Dwell In.

—ISAIAH 58:12

Since we have talked about living foods today, let's talk about other ways to bring life into our spirits and our families. The verse we've highlighted today comes from Isaiah 58, often called the fasting chapter of the Bible because it defines the kind of fast God will honor. In verse 12, we read that fasting has the power to restore and bring reconciliation. Perhaps your loved ones are far from Christ, and, as a result, there has been a breakdown in your relationship with them. Through fasting, you can break the power of darkness that keeps your loved ones from experiencing the truth of the gospel, and God can restore and rebuild what the enemy has stolen. God has a plan for your family. He can bring the life of salvation into their hearts and can restore life in your relationship with them. If there are people or situations in your life that need the miraculous restorative power of God's Spirit, list them here.

_____

_____

_____

Now, let's pray for those people and situations. You can pray the following prayer or use your own words.

Dear Lord, I thank You that Your Word promises that You will restore what the enemy has taken from my life. I declare today that by the authority of Jesus in my life, I will no longer allow the enemy to steal from my health, my relationships, or my home. Bring the reconciliation power of Your Spirit into every situation, and may each person I encounter today be touched by Your love. In Jesus' name, amen.

RECORD YOUR THOUGHTS

Use the space provided to record anything God brings to your mind as you pray today.

_____

_____

_____

_____

DAY 6

MEAL SUGGESTIONS

Breakfast	Snack	Lunch	Dinner
Brown Rice Grits* (page 145)	Roasted Red Pepper Wraps (page 153)	Cucumber and Onion Salad (page 161)	Veggie Pot Pie (page 173)

FOCUS THOUGHT

Humble fasting before God is awesomely powerful and can turn an entire nation around.

YOUR DAILY PRESCRIPTION FOR HEALTH

Choosing your foods is the first step toward a health-first lifestyle, but the way you prepare those foods is just as important. Deep-frying causes food (french fries, chicken, chicken strips, onion rings, etc.) to soak up free radicals and lose nutrients. There are much healthier ways to cook your food. Stir-frying is a good method since the food is cooked so briefly that it retains most of its nutrients. Simply use a small amount of organic extra-virgin olive, coconut, or macadamia nut oil. Grilling is also generally safe. Use a propane gas grill in place of charcoal or mesquite, which contain dangerous toxins. Place the vegetable or meat rack as high as possible away from the flame. If meat cooks over a flame, the fat drips off the meat and into the fire, which turns it into steam. The pesticides in the fat char into the meat so that even greater amounts of carcinogens are formed. Avoid charring meat since it contains a chemical called benzopyrene, which is a highly carcinogenic substance. Scrape or cut off the char.

YOUR DAILY SPIRITUAL JOURNEY

And as day was about to dawn, Paul implored them all to take food, saying, "Today is the fourteenth day you have waited and continued without food, and eaten nothing. Therefore I urge you to take nourishment, for this is for your survival, since not a hair will fall from the head of any of you."

—ACTS 27:33–34

Fasting is a biblical practice that gets results. God expects you to fast. It will help accomplish His purpose in your life. It is a wonderful way to crucify our own wants and desires and focus on the things that are important to

God. It also brings God's deliverance into situations that have brought you continuous trouble. If you are in the midst of trials, be encouraged: God has not forgotten you. He promised the sailors in Acts 27 that not a single hair would fall from their heads. He knows exactly where you are and what you need. Believe Him for a breakthrough in your situation as you humble yourself through fasting today. Use this space to describe the stressful situation you are facing today, this week, or this month.

_____

_____

_____

Here's a sample prayer:

Father, Your Word says that whatever a man sows, he will also reap. I claim that for my health today. As I sow good health by eating and cooking in healthy ways, I trust that You will be faithful to produce good health in my life. I also claim the principle of sowing and reaping for the troublesome situations that the enemy has used to try and hinder me. As I sow Your Word and Your presence into my life, I expect to reap breakthroughs for Your glory. In Jesus' name, amen.

RECORD YOUR THOUGHTS

Use the space provided to write down what you feel God is laying on your heart during this time.

_____

_____

_____

DAY 7

DR. COLBERT'S CLEANSING AND DETOX FAST

MEAL SUGGESTIONS

Breakfast	Snack	Lunch	Dinner
Breakfast Sweet Potatoes and Toasted Bagel (pages 145, 146)	Banana-Almond Delight (page 153)	Greek Salad (page 161)	Garden Variety Soup (page 173)

FOCUS THOUGHT

Tap water may contain heavy metals, pesticides, bacteria, other microbes, chlorine, fluoride, aluminum, and many other chemicals and toxins. It's best not to drink tap water or use it for cooking.

YOUR DAILY PRESCRIPTION FOR HEALTH

Many people choose to drink tap water; however, this is not a wise choice. One government report identified more than two thousand chemicals in our drinking water.[4] However, most water-testing facilities can only perform tests for approximately thirty or forty chemicals. Municipal treatment plants neither detect nor remove most chemicals from the water supply. The underground aquifers that feed city water supplies may catch runoff from dump sites, landfills, and even underground storage tanks. Sooner or later anything we bury, spray, emit, or flush finds its way into our drinking water. Tap water is good for watering lawns, washing clothes, and flushing toilets, but not for drinking or cooking. If you have been drinking tap water or beverages made from tap water (iced tea, coffee, etc.), I strongly recommend that you either purchase a water filter or pure, bottled water. For more information on this topic, watch for my upcoming book *The Seven Pillars of Health.*[5]

YOUR DAILY SPIRITUAL JOURNEY

The Lord will…satisfy your soul in drought, and strengthen your bones.
—ISAIAH 58:11

Another benefit of fasting in Isaiah 58 is mental, physical, and spiritual refreshment. The Bible also tells us in Isaiah 40:31 that when we wait on the Lord, it renews our strength. Like streams of pure, clean water flowing down from heaven, God's Spirit can wash over us and make us fresh and new. Allow His refreshing to wash away weariness, worry, and spiritual dryness today. As you spend time in His presence, wait upon Him in silence and allow Him to renew your strength.

Here's a simple prayer for you to pray:

Dear Lord, I receive Your refreshing today. I ask that Your Spirit would burst forth in my life like springs of living water. I thirst for more of You and ask You to fill me to overflowing today. With Job I can say, "Lord, I have treasured the words of Your mouth more than my necessary food" (Job 23:12). In Jesus' name, amen.

RECORD YOUR THOUGHTS

Use the space provided to express your thirst for more of God in your life.

_____

_____

_____

_____

DR. COLBERT'S CLEANSING AND DETOX FAST

DAY 8

MEAL SUGGESTIONS

Breakfast	Snack	Lunch	Dinner
Hot and Creamy Cereal* (page 146)	Hummus* on spelt or Ezekiel bagel (page 154)	Quick and Tasty Black Beans, Mexican Rice,* and Fresh Salsa (pages 162, 186)	Lemon-Basil Pasta Tossed With Broccoli and Zucchini (page 174)

FOCUS THOUGHT

When you sit down to eat, take time to thank God and to meditate on all His goodness and provision. Release any negative emotions, bless the food, and then begin to eat.

YOUR DAILY PRESCRIPTION FOR HEALTH

Make dining your most pleasant times of the day—especially dinner. It should be a time to slow down, relax, and gather with family and friends to enjoy the food and fellowship. The atmosphere at mealtime should be peaceful, pleasant, and joyful. Turn off the television; don't even watch sporting events, the news, or movies. Begin your meal with a blessing and then pause and consider how thankful you are. Always keep the conversation pleasant, and never use the dinner table as a time to reprimand your children or discuss stressful topics for yourself or your children. Never argue or complain at the table, but instead choose to compliment, encourage, tell funny or entertaining stories, and simply relax and fellowship with one another.

At restaurants I commonly hear families arguing, complaining, and fussing with one another. Realize that when you are stressed, you can't digest as well and are more prone to develop heartburn, indigestion, bloating, and gas.

If you are angry, upset, or just irritated, then wait to eat. When families sit down to a meal together, especially dinner, parents are given a chance to reconnect with their children.

Make it a point to create a pleasant environment at meal time and if arguments or complaints begin, redirect the conversation to wholesome, pleasant topics.

YOUR DAILY SPIRITUAL JOURNEY

Those from among you shall build the old waste places; you shall raise up the foundations of many generations.

—ISAIAH 58:12

In Isaiah 58, we see that there is a promise to raise up the foundations of many generations through fasting. Is there strife in your family? The Bible says that both blessings and curses can be passed from one generation to the next. We often hear the term *generational curses* to refer to this. Generational curses can be physical (as in the predisposition for illness and disease), but they can also be character traits. Are there generational curses of anger, unkindness, or disrespecting others that need to be broken in your family? List the behaviors you may have learned while growing up that you want to break before they are passed on to your children.

_____

_____

_____

Lord, I realize that my speech needs to be a reflection of Your Spirit at work within me. Let my speech be full of grace. I renounce any generational curse that would cause me to use words that tear others down. Fill my mouth with words that will bring life to those around me and build them up. In Jesus' name, amen.

RECORD YOUR THOUGHTS

Use the space provided to record your thoughts and prayer requests.

_____

_____

_____

DAY 9

DR. COLBERT'S CLEANSING AND DETOX FAST

MEAL SUGGESTIONS

Breakfast	Snack	Lunch	Dinner
Breakfast Tacos (page 146)	Spelt tortilla chips and Black Bean Dip* (page 154)	Incredible Summer Slaw* (page 163)	Brown Rice Risotto* and Zucchini Carpacio* (pages 175, 174)

FOCUS THOUGHT

Don't overeat. Only eat until you are satisfied and no more. Overeating places an enormous added burden on your liver and detoxification pathways.

YOUR DAILY PRESCRIPTION FOR HEALTH

The main reason many Americans are obese is simply gluttony, and Christians are no exception. A study from Purdue University found that religious people are more likely to be overweight than are nonreligious people.[6]

If you tend to be an overeater, here are some pointers that can help. Fill your plate in the kitchen and place it on the table rather than serving yourself at the table. Chew your food slowly (each bite should be chewed thirty times), and rest between bites. Set your fork down between bites. Give your stomach a chance to find out how full it is before you give it more. It generally takes twenty minutes for the brain to inform you that you are full or satisfied, so slow down while eating. A deep breath at the end of a meal is generally a sign that your body is satisfied. Plan a walk right after dinner. When you dine out, take half of your order home for the next day, or split the meal with your spouse.

YOUR DAILY SPIRITUAL JOURNEY

Or do you not know that your body is the temple of the Holy Spirit who is in you, whom you have from God, and you are not your own? For you were bought at a price; therefore glorify God in your body and in your spirit, which are God's.
—1 CORINTHIANS 6:19-20

Gluttony, or undisciplined eating, is a spiritual and emotional problem first and foremost; it's a dietary problem second. Gluttony is simply a lack of temperance. In all of my years of medical practice, I have treated thousands of patients with a weight problem, and almost always the root cause is emotional. They have usually tried many different diets and failed. The moment they mess up and eat the wrong food, they feel guilty and ashamed. If you fit this description, take a moment to write down your experiences in the space provided.

_____

_____

_____

It is worth mentioning that you don't have to be overweight to be a glutton. If your weight is normal but you constantly gorge yourself on every unhealthy food your flesh desires, you are just as out of control as any overweight person. Remember, God looks on the heart and sees the lack of discipline in your life.

Break out of unhealthy, undisciplined eating by loving, accepting, and forgiving yourself. Realize that no one is going to restrain your appetite—not even God. Only you can do that. You must begin to make the right choices in both food and drink. Spend a few minutes thinking about changes you need to make in your eating and drinking habits. List them here.

_____

_____

_____

Now let's pray for the power to break free from gluttony.

Dear Lord, as I continue to fast, I am encouraged to realize that it will cause others to see You in me. As Your Spirit gives me power to break free from undisciplined eating habits, I ask that more of Your character and power will flow through my life. I cannot break these habits in my own strength. I receive Your strength to exercise temperance and break free from gluttony for Your glory. In Jesus' name, amen.

RECORD YOUR THOUGHTS

Use the space provided to write about your goal to become more disciplined and the ways you think God will help you.

_____

_____

_____

DAY 10

DR. COLBERT'S CLEANSING AND DETOX FAST

MEAL SUGGESTIONS

Breakfast	Snack	Lunch	Dinner
Pecan Quinoa* (page 147)	Bruschetta (page 154)	Rainbow Fruit Salad (page 163)	Five Bean Soup (page 175)

FOCUS THOUGHT

You are what you eat—especially when it comes to your physical body. And what you eat will make all the difference in maintaining, strengthening, and detoxifying your liver.

YOUR DAILY PRESCRIPTION FOR HEALTH

Everything you put in your mouth has the potential to produce life or death. Consistently eating the wrong foods will eventually cause poor health and disease. All foods are not created equal. Living foods were created for our consumption. They exist in a raw or close-to-raw state. Living foods include fruit, vegetables, whole grains, seeds, and nuts. No chemicals have been added. They have not been bleached or chemically altered. Living foods are plucked, harvested, and squeezed, not processed, packaged, and put on a shelf.

If you want to be healthy, vibrant, and energetic, then you must begin to choose to eat more living foods. If you can eat at least 50 percent of your food as living food, you are much more likely to be healthy and resistant to most diseases.

YOUR DAILY SPIRITUAL JOURNEY

I have set before you life and death, blessing and cursing; therefore choose life, that both you and your descendants may live.

—DEUTERONOMY 30:19

This verse records a challenge Moses gave to the Israelites. It shows us how our choices affect the lives of the generations who follow after us. On Day 8, we talked about generational curses, but today, we're looking at "generational choices." Ask the Holy Spirit to reveal choices you have made that do not promote spiritual, emotional, or physical life or well-being. Do you now realize that these choices are not passing on healthy habits to your children? What choices will you make now to bring life and health to your family?

_____

_____

_____

How do you plan to implement change and create healthy, life-giving habits for the next generation in your household? Spend a few minutes thinking and praying before you write your answers. God may lay on your heart different ways to bring about change that you might not think of on your own.

_____

_____

_____

Now, make it a matter of prayer:

Dear Lord, I choose life today. I choose Your precious eternal life for me and my household, but I also choose an abundant life of health, prosperity, peace, and joy. Show me today any area of my life where my choices are not in line with the life-giving principles of Your Word. Empower me through Your Spirit to obey Your voice so that I may experience Your life and share it with others. In Jesus' name, amen.

RECORD YOUR THOUGHTS

Use the space provided to write anything God has revealed to you about your choices.

_____

_____

_____

_____

DAY 11

MEAL SUGGESTIONS

Breakfast	Snack	Lunch	Dinner
Banana Nut Cereal (page 147)	Nachos (page 155)	Avocado Salad* (page 164)	Mediterranean Pasta* and Italian Greens (page 176)

FOCUS THOUGHT

Wisdom is a pathway that God has given us to walk upon. When we choose to walk in wisdom, the benefits to our lives and health are limitless.

YOUR DAILY PRESCRIPTION FOR HEALTH

As an antioxidant, green tea is two hundred times more powerful than vitamin E and five hundred times more powerful than vitamin C. Green tea is believed to block the effect of cancer-causing chemicals. It also activates detoxification enzymes in the liver, which helps defend your body against cancer. For detoxification purposes, I recommend one cup of organic green tea two to three times a day. If you prefer, you may take green tea in capsule form. (See Appendix B.)

As you can imagine by now, antioxidants are extremely important in this vital work of your liver. Glutathione is one of the most important and abundant antioxidants in the body. The liver is a hotbed of free-radical activity, and adequate levels of glutathione are essential to prevent damage by free radicals. The amino acid NAC (N-acetyl cysteine) is converted in the body to glutathione. Also the powerful antioxidant DHLA (dihydrolipoic acid) is able to quench every known free radical that occurs in living tissue, both water and fat soluble. It regenerates vitamin C, vitamin E, CoQ_{10}, and glutathione. Another form of lipoic acid called R-form alpha-lipoic acid is also an excellent supplement. (See Appendix B.)

YOUR DAILY SPIRITUAL JOURNEY

Therefore do not be unwise, but understand what the will of the Lord is.
—EPHESIANS 5:17

You may have days where you wonder about your purpose and whether you even have one. Fasting and prayer can reveal God's purpose to you and bring focus to your life. You don't have to be in the dark when it comes to knowing His will for the future. You can know that you are following His path. He has an assignment for you, and He will reveal it to you. If you have any thoughts or questions about God's will and purpose for your life, take a moment to write them down here.

_____

_____

_____

Now, spend a few minutes in prayer, asking God to reveal His will to you. You can pray this prayer or a similar one in your own words.

Dear Lord, I trust You to lead and guide me so that I will follow Your path for my life. Direct my decisions today concerning my future, my family, and my finances. Everything I have is Yours to use for Your glory—my body, my gifts and talents, my money and possessions. I stand in faith, expecting that You will show me the good plans You have for me, according to Jeremiah 29:11. In Jesus' name, amen.

As Dr. Bob Rodgers says in his book *The 21-Day Fast*, "Every assignment has a birthplace. Let this...fast be the birthplace where you find your true mission in life."[7]

RECORD YOUR THOUGHTS

If you sense God giving you an "assignment" or revealing His will for your life, write it down in the space provided, along with today's date.

_____

_____

_____

DAY 12

DR. COLBERT'S CLEANSING AND DETOX FAST

MEAL SUGGESTIONS

Breakfast	Snack	Lunch	Dinner
Egg-less French Toast (page 148)	Pepitas (page 155)	Summer Garden Salad* (page 164)	Veggie Shepherd's Pie (page 177)

FOCUS THOUGHT

If you want an easy, natural way to boost your self-image, build your confidence, and increase your energy, determine to exercise at least twenty minutes a day, three to four days a week.

YOUR DAILY PRESCRIPTION FOR HEALTH

I recommend that to ensure a healthy, fasted lifestyle, you plan to include a good exercise program. Many toxins can be expelled simply through perspiration as you give your body the exercise it needs. Exercise is also an antidote for stress, helping to relax tight muscles and release the tension of the day.

Regular exercise improves heart health, lung function, circulation, and blood pressure. Exercise can actually decrease fatigue as it relaxes your muscles and reduces stress. As you exercise, your body also releases endorphins, which are natural antidepressants and pain relievers, which results in your feeling better after you exercise.

Aerobic exercise helps to calm your body as well as your mind by releasing tension. During your fast, it is best to keep this exercise light so that you do not become overly tired. You may want to get together with friends for a walk, tennis, or a bike ride. Choose to exercise in a way that is enjoyable to you, and you will be more likely to succeed in it.

YOUR DAILY SPIRITUAL JOURNEY

...to loose the bonds of wickedness, to undo the heavy burdens?
—ISAIAH 58:6

In the same way that light exercise during a fast relieves tension and stress, spiritual fasting can relieve us from burdens that regular prayer cannot break through. The Bible uses words such as *burden* or *yoke* to describe those things that keep us from experiencing freedom in Christ. They hold us captive, and our limited human strength is not enough to break us loose.

But in Isaiah 58:6, we learn that fasting has the power to undo heavy burdens and problems that seem too great to bear. What circumstances in your life have become burdensome for you—finances? Stresses of everyday life? Chronic illness? Legal problems? Taxes? Difficult neighbors, co-workers, or family members? Write about the areas where you need a breakthrough in the space provided.

_____

_____

_____

Dear Lord, I believe that You have set me free and that, therefore, I am free indeed! I stand in faith that You will move on my behalf to change circumstances in my life and set me free from burdens and strongholds that have held me captive. I lay down those situations that I have tried to carry even though You never intended for me to carry them. No matter how hopeless the situation, I will no longer try to handle it in my own strength, but I will wait to see Your hand of deliverance at work in my life. In Jesus' name, amen.

RECORD YOUR THOUGHTS

Use the space provided to record the burdens you sense God is releasing from your life today.

_____

_____

_____

DAY 13

DR. COLBERT'S CLEANSING AND DETOX FAST

MEAL SUGGESTIONS

Breakfast	Snack	Lunch	Dinner
Oatmeal Waffles (page 148)	Un-Caviar (page 156)	Grilled Mushroom Salad with Sesame Ginger Dressing* (pages 164, 185)	Sun-Dried Tomato Pasta* and salad with Garlic Herb Dressing* (pages 177, 184)

FOCUS THOUGHT

Don't eat when you're stressed. Before you pick up your fork, take a brief moment to relax a bit by taking five to ten slow, deep abdominal breaths. It's extremely important.

YOUR DAILY PRESCRIPTION FOR HEALTH

The efficiency of your GI tract is being challenged every day. One of those challenges comes from a deficiency of those incredibly powerful digestive juices. If you are over fifty years old, you may be among the many middle-aged individuals who begin to experience a reduction in the hydrochloric acid that is so essential to digestion. When the levels of this acid become depleted, digestive problems follow.

If stress plays a major role in your life, you probably don't need me to tell you that it affects digestion. It's not unusual for stressed-out individuals to have stomach medications strewed all around their workplace and home. If you are stressed, you are probably not only deficient in hydrochloric acid, but you may be deficient in pancreatic enzymes as well. The lack of these vital pancreatic enzymes causes poor digestion of proteins, fats, and carbohydrates. When this happens, bits of partially digested food can putrefy and eventually lead to bacterial overgrowth in the small intestines, food allergies, leaky gut (increased intestinal permeability), irritable bowel syndrome, and so forth.

YOUR DAILY SPIRITUAL JOURNEY

You shall be like a watered garden, and like a spring of water, whose waters do not fail.

—ISAIAH 58:11

The watered garden and unfailing spring in Isaiah 58:11 are similes for prosperity. This passage tells us that God's blessings will not fail. They will not end. We can look to Him as our source and our provider, and He will rain down His provisions upon us and quench the dry surface of our hearts. Stress will evaporate. Curses will be broken. Needs and, yes, even desires will be met.

During these days of fasting, pray that your desires would be the desires of God. Pray that His will for your life will be reflected in the desires of your heart. As you take a spiritual inventory of your life, you need to let go of your old ways of thinking and unhealthy habits, and take hold of God's plan for your life. As you turn away from sin and trust God with your whole heart, He will pour out blessings upon you that you can't even contain. In the space provided, list the desires of your heart that you feel line up with God's plan for your life.

_____

_____

_____

Now, let's spend some time in prayer.

Dear Lord, I know that You said You are able to do above and beyond anything that I can ever ask or think. I believe that You are already working to bestow blessings upon me as I seek to know the desires of Your heart. With each new blessing, may I be made more faithful, and may I never forget to praise You and thank You for all that You have done and continue to do in my life. In Jesus' name, amen.

RECORD YOUR THOUGHTS

In the space provided, record what you sense God is laying on your heart during this time of prayer.

_____

_____

_____

_____

DR. COLBERT'S CLEANSING AND DETOX FAST

DAY 14

MEAL SUGGESTIONS

Breakfast	Snack	Lunch	Dinner
Crispy Brown Rice Flakes (page 148)	Veggie Panini (page 156)	Sautéed Baby Spinach* and Pasta Primavera* (page 165)	Country Cabbage Soup* and Sesame Spelt Bread* (pages 178, 182)

FOCUS THOUGHT

If poor lifestyle choices have brought disease into your body, don't condemn yourself; God does not condemn you. Begin making better choices based upon godly wisdom.

YOUR DAILY PRESCRIPTION FOR HEALTH

Fiber is fantastic for your healthy GI tract. It acts like a broom, sweeping the colon lining, eliminating the toxins, and binding toxins and bile so that they cannot be reabsorbed back into your body. All of this activity is critically important in preventing disease. High-fiber diets also reduce the level of circulating estrogens by binding them and preventing them from being reabsorbed and recirculated through the liver.

Most of the chemicals that have been detoxified by the liver are contained in the bile, which is then dumped into the intestinal tract. This, as you know, is a major part of your body's detoxification process. But if your GI tract doesn't have enough fiber or is constipated, then much of that toxic bile will be reabsorbed back into your body. That's why it's so important to get plenty of fiber every day through your diet and to supplement with fiber regularly as well so that the toxins in your body will be bound and excreted. This will dramatically reduce your body's toxic burden.

YOUR DAILY SPIRITUAL JOURNEY

I proclaimed a fast, so that we might humble ourselves before our God and ask him for a safe journey for us and our children, with all our possessions.

—EZRA 8:21, NIV

Here's the story behind today's Scripture verse. The Jewish nation had been held in captivity in Persia for centuries. When freedom finally came, Ezra, a priest, was given permission to return to Jerusalem to rebuild the magnificent temple. The trip to Jerusalem was very dangerous. Ezra needed guidance and protection to lead the great caravan of thousands of defenseless Jews back to their home city. So, he proclaimed a fast for protection, security, and direction from God.

The traveling Jews returned to Jerusalem in safety with all of their possessions intact. Once again, the Bible reports powerful spiritual results were obtained through fasting. What situations do you need to seek God's protection and guidance for today? Describe them in the space provided.

_____

_____

_____

Dear Lord, come and sweep away the cobwebs of disbelief from my heart. Reveal the way that I should go, and grant me the boldness and faith to step out and walk that path, regardless of what others say or do. Grant me protection from the enemy and those who would seek to harm or hinder me. In Jesus' name, amen.

RECORD YOUR THOUGHTS

Use the space provided to record any guidance or leading from God that you sense in your heart today.

_____

_____

_____

DAY 15

DR. COLBERT'S CLEANSING AND DETOX FAST

MEAL SUGGESTIONS

Breakfast	Snack	Lunch	Dinner
Oatmeal Waffles and Green Apple Compote* (pages 148, 149)	Tomato Cucumber Relish* (page 164)	Cleansing Cabbage Salad (page 165)	Minestrone* (page 178)

FOCUS THOUGHT

Digestion actually begins when your brain signals that your body needs food. When you start thinking about the minestrone you are making for dinner, your brain signals your digestive tract to begin producing the necessary enzymes and components for digestion.

YOUR DAILY PRESCRIPTION FOR HEALTH

Imagine that your skin suddenly turned to glass so that you could see everything going on inside of you. You would quickly see that your intestinal tract is, stated simply, a long, winding tube. As a matter of fact, it is a continuous tube that's more than twenty feet long. It connects your entire digestive system together. Your food enters the tube on one end and exits on the other.

In between, your food undergoes a miracle of processing. The mouth starts the process and connects with the esophagus. The esophagus connects with the stomach. The stomach connects with the small intestines. The small intestines connect with the large intestines, and the large intestines connect to the rectum and finally end at the anus. If digestion and elimination proceed smoothly and unhindered and you consume enough water and fiber, then toxins are eliminated daily, and good health is achieved.

YOUR DAILY SPIRITUAL JOURNEY

So it was, when Ahab heard those words, that he…fasted and lay in sackcloth, and went about mourning. And the word of the Lord came to Elijah the Tishbite, saying, "See how Ahab has humbled himself before Me? Because he has humbled himself before Me, I will not bring the calamity in his days."

—1 KINGS 21:27–29

Fasting enables us to receive God's mercy and grace. In the scripture above, we see that God withheld judgment from Ahab because he humbled himself through fasting. God's mercy and grace are available to you today. Whatever your situation, if you repent and humble yourself before God, He will be faithful and just to forgive you and place you in right standing with Him.

You may also use this time of fasting to ask for God's mercy upon our nation. Seek God on behalf of our country, and ask His forgiveness for the ungodly people we have become. Use the space provided to write the specific things that you sense God is leading you to repent of on behalf of our nation.

_____

_____

_____

Now take those things to God in prayer.

Dear Lord, You said that if Your people would humble themselves and pray, and turn from their wicked ways, that You would hear from heaven, forgive their sins, and heal their land. I ask You to do this in my home and in my country today. I receive Your mercy and grace and thank You that Your mercies are new every morning and that they never fail. In Jesus' name, amen.

RECORD YOUR THOUGHTS

Use the space provided to write about the mercy and grace of God in your life, your family, your community, or the nation.

_____

_____

_____

_____

DAY 16

DR. COLBERT'S CLEANSING AND DETOX FAST

MEAL SUGGESTIONS

Breakfast	Snack	Lunch	Dinner
Fresh Berries With Lemon-Coconut Sauce and sprouted English muffin (page 149)	Cucumbers With Lime (page 157)	Field Greens Salad* and Lemon Grape Seed Oil Dressing* (pages 166, 185)	Tortilla Soup and Quick Guacamole* (pages 179, 186)

FOCUS THOUGHT

When you go on a water-only fast, mechanisms in your brain will eventually signal your body that you are starving even if you are not. Therefore, your body goes into a survival state to try and hold on to all the calories it gets.

YOUR DAILY PRESCRIPTION FOR HEALTH

The strictest, most severe fast is a water-only fast. In general, I usually don't recommend this type of fasting. But for certain autoimmune diseases such as lupus and rheumatoid arthritis or for severe atherosclerosis such as severe coronary artery disease, the benefits of water-only fasting are powerful in select individuals. Nevertheless, you can also experience similar benefits for these diseases with juice fasting—it just takes longer. For most individuals, water-only fasting so weakens the body that working a full-time job while fasting is not possible. Juice fasting provides most of the benefits of water-only fasting without the unpleasant weakness and hunger that often accompany a water-only fast.

YOUR DAILY SPIRITUAL JOURNEY

Then you shall call, and the Lord will answer; you shall cry, and He will say, "Here I am."

—ISAIAH 58:9

Fasting draws us into God's presence. He reveals more of Himself to us when we humble ourselves and call on Him. Fasting allowed Moses to enter such a depth of God's presence that the very glory of God came upon him and radiated to everyone nearby.

God's presence brings God's power. Fasting and drawing near to God's presence enable us to touch the world around us with God's love and power. In fact, it was with fasting that the apostles in the first century sent out their missionaries to proclaim the message of Christ. (See Acts 13:2–3.) They realized that fasting is a tool to access God's power, which can in turn affect your spouse, your children, your extended family, your community, and even the world.

Write about the people or situations you want to influence with God's power through your fast.

_____

_____

_____

Lord, I thank You that I receive power when Your Holy Spirit comes upon me through fasting. Just as Moses was changed by encountering Your glory, I pray that as I draw nearer to You and experience Your presence during this time of fasting, it will change and empower me to be a witness to others of Your mercy, goodness, and love. In Jesus' name, amen.

RECORD YOUR THOUGHTS

Use the space provided to record your time with God in prayer today. Do you sense His power working in you to be a witness or catalyst for change to those around you? Write about it.

_____

_____

_____

DAY 17

DR. COLBERT'S CLEANSING AND DETOX FAST

MEAL SUGGESTIONS

Breakfast	Snack	Lunch	Dinner
Cantaloupe-Berry Delight and spelt bagel (page 149)	Veggie-Nut Bars (page 157)	Whipped Butternut Squash* and Broiled Tomato Sandwich (page 166)	Butterbean Soup and Garlic Bread* (pages 179, 183)

FOCUS THOUGHT

Isn't it interesting that God placed beautiful colors of red, blue, and purple in different fruits and vegetables that provide protection from most diseases and actually keep you looking younger?

YOUR DAILY PRESCRIPTION FOR HEALTH

Flavonoids are a group of powerful phytonutrients. They are found in red, purple, and blue plant pigments, especially blackberries, blueberries, cherries, and grapes. Flavonoids can keep your skin looking younger. This is because they play an enormous role in the formation and repair of collagen. Collagen is the main structural protein in the body, and it is also the most abundant protein found in your body. It actually holds the cells and tissues of your body together. Collagen tends to degenerate with age and slowly collapse, which is why our skin begins to sag as we get older. However, the flavonoids found in berries, cherries, grapes, and a host of other fruits and vegetables help to maintain the integrity of your skin's collagen. Therefore, it helps to keep your skin's collagen from degenerating and collapsing with age. By simply juicing berries and grapes every day, you can get enough flavonoids to nourish your skin's collagen and slow down the aging process.

YOUR DAILY SPIRITUAL JOURNEY

Then your light shall break forth like the morning.

—ISAIAH 58:8

Revelation and a deeper sensitivity to spiritual things come when people fast. When Daniel fasted for twenty-one days in Daniel 10, the angel Gabriel came and revealed the future to him. When Cornelius fasted in Acts 10, God told him to send for Peter, while at the same time, as Peter fasted, God gave him a vision to go to the Gentiles and preach the gospel.

As you fast and pray, ask God to bring new revelation to you. Ask Him to reveal His plan for your unsaved family members and friends. List their names here, along with anything you sense He is revealing to you about them.

_____

_____

_____

Dear Lord, reveal Yourself to me. I ask for a deeper understanding of who You are and what You are doing in my life and in the lives of those around me. Cleanse my heart from the things that hinder my prayers, and cause me to rejoice over the things that fill Your heart with joy. As my focus becomes clearer, show me a fresh revelation of things to come. In Jesus' name, amen.

RECORD YOUR THOUGHTS

Use the space provided to record any further revelation you feel God is showing you during your prayer time today.

_____

_____

_____

DR. COLBERT'S CLEANSING AND DETOX FAST

DAY 18

MEAL SUGGESTIONS

Breakfast	Snack	Lunch	Dinner
Ginger Fruit Mix and millet toast (page 150)	Peach Salsa (page 158)	Butternut Tomato Soup (page 167)	Mushroom Barley Soup (page 180)

FOCUS THOUGHT

Are you listening to your body? Do you understand what it is trying to tell you? How is your physical body responding to my fasting program?

YOUR DAILY PRESCRIPTION FOR HEALTH

The main causes of increased intestinal permeability (microscopic openings or holes in the small intestine caused by inflammation) are food allergies, food sensitivities, and, many times, antibiotic usage. Common food allergies include allergies to egg, dairy products, corn, soy, yeast, wheat, and other grains such as rye, barley, and oats. The main protein that people are sensitive to in these grains is gluten, which is found in breads, crackers, pasta, all kinds of flour (such as rye, barley, wheat and oat flour), gravies, many soups, bread crumbs, pies, and cakes.

Increased intestinal permeability is usually present in the following diseases: chronic fatigue, fibromyalgia, migraine headaches, eczema, hives, psoriasis, Crohn's disease, ulcerative colitis, celiac disease, rheumatoid arthritis, lupus, schizophrenia, autism, and attention-deficit hyperactivity disorder. If you suspect this might be an issue for you, this liver detoxification and fasting program should benefit you. If you are sensitive to gluten, select another form of grain for your daily diet, such as brown rice bread, millet bread, quinoa, kamut, or amaranth. Buckwheat is also gluten-free, so you can still have buckwheat pancakes.

YOUR DAILY SPIRITUAL JOURNEY

Then your light shall break forth like the morning, your healing shall spring forth speedily; and your righteousness shall go before you.

—ISAIAH 58:8

I believe fasting releases God's power in your life. There are many instances recorded in Scripture of God's supernatural intervention in individual lives and in nations when His people humbled themselves through prayer and fasting. Moses fasted for forty days as he waited in God's presence on the mountain and received the law of God for Israel. Daniel fasted and prayed for twenty-one days for his nation, seeking God to fulfill His promise to deliver them from captivity, which was accomplished. The early church "ministered to the Lord and fasted" (Acts 13:1–3). The spiritual power released through fasting will enable us to touch the world around us with God's love and power.

Describe a situation in your life that needs God's power.

_____

_____

_____

There is also a scriptural promise of a release of God's healing power through fasting, as we see in our verse from Isaiah 58. This type of fasting involves more than simply denying ourselves certain foods for a time; it involves a change in attitude and showing compassion to the needy as well. Releasing the healing power of God in our lives as we subdue the destructive appetites of the flesh is a wonderful benefit of spiritual fasting. Claim God's healing power for your life or someone you know by praying this prayer.

Dear Lord, I believe that my healing (or my loved one's healing) will spring forth speedily as my body recovers from any disease or traumatic accident. As I humble myself through fasting, I enter Your presence and touch the hem of Your garment, and by Your stripes I am healed. In Jesus' name, amen.

RECORD YOUR THOUGHTS

Use the space provided to record anything you sense God is laying on your heart about healing today.

_____

_____

_____

DAY 19

DR. COLBERT'S CLEANSING AND DETOX FAST

MEAL SUGGESTIONS

Breakfast	Snack	Lunch	Dinner
Fresh Fruit Cup and Ezekiel bread (page 150)	Frosted Grapes (page 158)	Cauliflower-Pea Soup (page 166)	Beverly's Black Bean Soup (page 180)

FOCUS THOUGHT

Each lifestyle choice that you and I make leads us down a pathway—to peace and joy or to stress and hardship. Be sure you know where your choices are leading you.

YOUR DAILY PRESCRIPTION FOR HEALTH

Milk thistle extract, known as silymarin, is one of the most powerful protectors of the liver against free-radical damage. It also protects the liver from many different extremely toxic chemicals, including the poisonous mushroom amanita phalloides, which is actually fatal in 40 percent of the people who ingest it.

Milk thistle prevents the depletion of the powerful antioxidant glutathione. Since vast amounts of glutathione can be expended in the detoxification process, it can lead to glutathione depletion. Milk thistle will prevent this depletion during detoxification. Milk thistle can actually raise the level of glutathione in the liver up to 35 percent.

Milk thistle is one of the most important antioxidant to take during the detoxification fasting program. The best form of milk thistle that I have found is a product called Silybin Phytosome. I recommend one capsule two times a day, or more if desired. (See Appendix B.)

YOUR DAILY SPIRITUAL JOURNEY

...to let the oppressed go free, and that you break every yoke?

—ISAIAH 58:6

Sexual addictions are some of the most difficult addictions to break. But fasting helps break the power of sexual addictions like pornography, homosexuality, masturbation, fornication, adultery, and lust. If you or someone you know is bound in any form of sexual addiction, make this the focus of your prayer time today. Describe the situation in the space provided.

_____

_____

_____

Dear Lord, I know that You can break every addiction and heal every broken relationship for Your glory. Father, right now, I claim that those things that the enemy is intending to use for evil You will turn around and use for good as we repent and consecrate our lives as holy unto You. I break the yoke of sexual addiction over myself and my loved ones. Bring Your deliverance, peace, and healing to everyone involved. May faithfulness operate where the lust of the flesh once abounded. In Jesus' name, amen.

RECORD YOUR THOUGHTS

Use the space provided to write about any thoughts that have come to your mind about addictions as you have spent time in prayer today.

_____

_____

_____

DR. COLBERT'S CLEANSING AND DETOX FAST

DAY 20

MEAL SUGGESTIONS

Breakfast	Snack	Lunch	Dinner
Mixed Berry Compote* and Buckwheat Pancakes (pages 150, 145)	No-Bake Granola (page 158)	Hacienda Pinto Beans* and Sweet Potato Salad* (pages 167, 168)	Fat-Burning Soup (page 181)

FOCUS THOUGHT

If you take over-the-counter medicines, consider more natural ways to treat your various medical conditions, such as nutrients, herbs, and homeopathics. However, you should never go off of medications that you need without consulting your doctor.

YOUR DAILY PRESCRIPTION FOR HEALTH

Few people ever consider that the health of their bodies is based upon a delicate natural acid and alkaline balance. Nevertheless, this balance is essential to your body's ability to detoxify successfully. When all your body gets is the standard American diet, your tissues become more acidic than nature intended—upsetting this delicate balance. If you would like to know how acidic your body is, you can find out very easily by simply purchasing some pH strips at the drugstore or health food store. Collect the first morning urine and dip a pH strip into it. It will indicate your urine's pH level with a change of color. The urinary pH usually indicates the pH of the tissues. The change of color can then be matched to a numerical reading. A card is included in the pH paper that correlates a color to a pH number. Most people will have a pH test reading of about 5.0, which means their bodies are very acidic. It should be between 6.8 and 7.0. Close enough doesn't count. Even though five is only two points less than seven, a pH of 5.0 is actually a hundred times more acidic than a pH of 7.0.

A healthy stomach has a pH between 1.5 and 3.0 due to hydrochloric acid, which is secreted by the stomach. Hydrocloric acid is strong enough to burn a hole through the carpet or to melt the iron in a nail. You can see how this powerful acid forms the first line of defense against bacteria, parasites, germs, and other microbes from our food.

YOUR DAILY SPIRITUAL JOURNEY

But seek first the kingdom of God and His righteousness, and all these things shall be added to you.

—MATTHEW 6:33

Just as your body must maintain a balanced pH, so you must find a balance in your spiritual life as well. Fasting can help bring this balance; it can help you get your priorities in the proper order. Jesus knew that the most important things in life are not what we have; they are who we are. That godly perspective brings balance to our lives. What areas have been out of balance for you? Have you been trying to control things that are out of your control? Describe the out-of-balance areas in your life.

_____

_____

_____

The key is to put Christ in His proper place of authority in your life. Then everything else will fall into place. Have you been worried about things that you need to give over to God? Allow Him to take those worries and cares from off of your shoulders and restore balance to your life.

Let's pray about it.

Dear Lord, I put Your kingdom first in my life. Help me to keep my commitment to serve You and be the person You've called me to be. You are my top priority. I thank You for this time of fasting that allows me to refocus my priorities and strengthen my desire to share Your love. I will not worry about the cares of this world, but keep my eyes focused on You. In Jesus' name, amen.

RECORD YOUR THOUGHTS

Use the space provided to record any out-of-balance areas of your life that you sense God is showing you during your prayer time today.

_____

_____

_____

DAY 21

DR. COLBERT'S CLEANSING AND DETOX FAST

MEAL SUGGESTIONS

Breakfast	Snack	Lunch	Dinner
Baked Apples (page 151)	Apple-Watermelon Smoothies (page 159)	Crock-Pot Bean Soup and Garlic Bread* (pages 168, 183)	Lentil Soup* (page 181)

FOCUS THOUGHT

Your amazing body is not only designed to detoxify itself but also to heal itself as well. And just as you can play a significant role in helping and supporting your body's own ability to detoxify itself, you can also do the same with healing.

YOUR DAILY PRESCRIPTION FOR HEALTH

As you gear up for the juice fast that makes up our final seven days, it's important to understand that the most important nutrients in fresh fruits and juices are the phytonutrients. Phytonutrients are simply plant-derived nutrients that contain powerful antioxidants and give fruits and vegetables their brilliant colors. These mighty plant nutrients prevent tumors and cancer, lower cholesterol, increase immune function, fight viruses, stimulate detoxification enzymes, prevent plaque buildup (which protects us against heart disease), and block the production of cancer-causing compounds.

Many of these phytonutrients are found in the pigments of the fruits and vegetables, such as the chlorophyll of green vegetables, the carotenes or carotenoids in orange fruits and vegetables, and the purple flavonoids in berries. One out of three Americans will at some time develop cancer in his or her lifetime.[8] Consuming adequate amounts of fruits and vegetables every day or in the form of juices is one of the best ways to protect your body from cancer and heart disease.

YOUR DAILY SPIRITUAL JOURNEY

And when He had come into the house, His disciples asked Him privately, "Why could we not cast [the evil spirit] out?" So He said to them, "This kind can come out by nothing but prayer and fasting."

—MARK 9:28–29

Whether you know it or not, you are in a spiritual battle between heaven and hell every day. Be willing to deny your physical desires and humbly seek the face of God during this time of fasting. Earnest, humble prayer will bring new strength to you and enable you to defeat the enemy and all of his demonic forces working to hinder your Christian walk. God will win the battle for you as you humble yourself in fasting and prayer.

There are some types of demonic activity that cannot be broken without fasting, as we see in today's scripture. If there is an area of your life where the spiritual warfare has been too great, now is the time to take authority in Jesus' name. With the added spiritual power of fasting, you will be able to break demonic oppression and set the captives free. Are there spiritual battles that need to be won in your life? List these issues, and commit to making them a matter of prayer during the remaining days of the fast.

_____

_____

Dear Lord, I know that my weapons are not carnal, but mighty through Your power. In the authority of Jesus, I can pull down strongholds and experience victory over evil. I pray for wisdom as I seek to do spiritual battle for breakthroughs in my life and in the lives of those I love. I thank You for giving me the victory. In Jesus' name, amen.

RECORD YOUR THOUGHTS

Use the space provided to record what God is laying on your heart during your prayer time today.

_____

_____

_____

CHAPTER 8

Detoxifying My Body With Juices

You stagger into the kitchen half-asleep, dragging the belt of your robe behind you like a long tail. Too groggy to speak, you pull your juicer out from a lower cabinet, plunk it on the counter, and reach for the apples, carrots, and other fruits and vegetables piled high in a giant bowl.

With the water running, you clean and chop the colorful ingredients of your first day's juice fast menu. In minutes, your juicer is whirring, spinning and extracting the elements of your brand-new, healthier, detoxified lifestyle.

It's done. You slowly, carefully touch your lips to the glass, wondering if you'll be able to drink this concoction you just made. But as you touch it to your tongue, you're amazed. It's more than delicious—it's delightful and refreshing. You had been willing to grit your teeth and endure this juicing program because you were convinced of its benefits to your health. But you never dreamed you would enjoy it so much!

I genuinely believe that you are going to find this fasting program more enjoyable, easier, and more rewarding than you ever expected. Not only that, but when you are through, your renewed energy and vitality will amaze you.

So let's get started with the juice fast portion of this detoxification program.

BEFORE YOU FAST

Before beginning the actual juice fasting portion of this program, you should have been following the diet to support your liver for twenty-one days. If you have completed the liver support diet, you are ready to detox. So, let's get started. Here are some pointers:

- As you begin, you should already have increased your intake of clean, pure water (not tap water) to two quarts a day. Continue drinking at least two quarts per day of pure water throughout the duration of your fast.

- During the fast, I do not recommend consuming vitamins. You should have taken a number of vitamins and minerals during the three weeks of your liver support diet. You must stop taking all of these supplements until your fasting period is over. After you complete the twenty-eight-day fasting program, you will need to resume taking a comprehensive multivitamin daily as a part of your new health-first lifestyle.

LET'S GET STARTED

To get started on your juice fast, you will want to purchase lots of fresh, organically grown vegetables and fruits. Organic produce is best because it is grown without pesticides and herbicides. If you don't think avoiding pesticides is an issue, you probably aren't aware that growers are free to use about four hundred different pesticides on crops. Each year in the United States, two billion pounds of pesticides and herbicides are sprayed on the food we eat.[1]

A study of government-collected data found pesticide residue on almost 75 percent of conventionally grown produce, but only 23 percent of organic fruits and vegetables were found to have residue.[2] So you can see that while purchasing organic produce doesn't mean your food will be completely pesticide free, it will greatly reduce the percentage of pesticide residue you ingest.

Since you are fasting to remove such chemicals, it's important to greatly reduce your intake of these chemicals during your fast. Organic produce can be found at many of the larger health food stores. There are even health food stores that are as large as some supermarkets, such as Whole Foods and Wild Oats. These have a wide variety of organic fruits and vegetables at a competitive price.

In addition, many of the larger supermarkets are beginning to stock organic produce as the public demands it. Our voices will be heard if we continue to ask the supermarket to carry organic products.

WHAT IF I CAN'T USE ORGANICS?

Organic produce tends to be more expensive, and it can be difficult to find. If you can't always use organics, then you must take special care to clean your fruits and vegetables to remove the waxes and chemicals. Here are some rules to remember when purchasing non-organic fruits and vegetables.

- *Look for thicker peels.* Bananas, oranges, tangerines, lemons, grapefruits, and watermelons are excellent fruits since they have a thicker peel and, therefore, fewer pesticides have soaked through into the fruit.

- *Watch thin peels.* If your produce has a thin peel, such as apples, pears, peaches, and nectarines, the pesticide has usually soaked through into the fruit. Based on an analysis of more than 100,000 U.S. government pesticide test results, researchers at the Environmental Working Group (EWG) concluded that among fruit, nectarines had the highest percentage of testing positive for pesticide residue.[3] You can reduce surface residue by peeling fruit before consumption, but nutrients and fiber may be lost in doing so. Therefore, I strongly recommend sticking to organic when buying produce with a thin peel.

- *Purchase domestic produce.* If you are unable to purchase organic produce, you can still reduce the amount of pesticides by purchasing produce grown in the United States. Produce grown in the States is generally safer than produce imported from other countries. Pesticides that have been banned in the United States are often exported to other countries such as Mexico. Many times, fruits and vegetables grown in these countries are sprayed with the banned pesticides and then exported to the United States.[4]

- *Wash off produce waxes.* You can purchase a natural, biodegradable cleanser from most health food stores, or simply wash your produce with a mild detergent such as pure castille soap from a health food store to remove waxes.

- *Use hydrogen peroxide to remove waxes and pesticides.* Soak the fruits and vegetables in a sink of cold water to which you have added 1 tablespoon of 35 percent, food-grade hydrogen peroxide for five to fifteen minutes. Then rinse them thoroughly with fresh water.

- *Use Clorox bleach.* Another good way to remove waxes and pesticides is to soak your produce in a sink half full of cold water with 1 teaspoon of Clorox bleach for five to fifteen minutes. Rinse the produce thoroughly for about three to five minutes.

CHOOSE A JUICER

There are many different types of juicers, and some are very expensive. You may start with an inexpensive juicer such as a Juice Man Junior juicer from Wal-Mart, which costs about $70. The Champion juicer is an excellent juicer and will usually last for decades. The Vita-Mix is a different type of juicer that looks more like a large blender. It is able to completely juice and liquefy the entire fruit or vegetable. This has the added benefit of providing the fiber in addition to the vitamins, minerals, antioxidants, enzymes, and phytonutrients. However, it is more expensive, usually costing over $400. I personally have all three types of juicers.

GUIDELINES FOR YOUR JUICE FAST

1. If you decide to go on a juice fast apart from the twenty-one day partial fast outlined in this book, you will want to prepare yourself by eating only fruits and vegetables the day before you begin your juice fast.
2. I strongly recommend that you begin your juice fast on the weekend. By doing so, you will be able to spend more time resting. If you experience any side effects such as fatigue, light-headedness, or a headache, it will probably not interfere with your job (since it is the weekend).
3. It's very important that you juice raw, fresh fruits and vegetables (preferably organic). Prepared juices are simply not the same. Fresh juice contains the living enzymes, phytonutrients, antioxidants, vitamins, and minerals. Bottled, canned, and processed juices have been pasteurized. Many of the phytonutrients and enzymes have been lost in the process.

4. Don't drink alcohol or soft drinks. During your fast, drink only juices and herbal teas. You may also sip gently warmed vegetable juice or vegetable broth. (Avoid microwaves since they destroy most of the phytonutrients, antioxidants, and enzymes.) Good teas include organic black, green, and herbal teas. Also, drink plenty of clean, pure water, about two quarts a day.

5. When drinking your specially prepared juices, sip them slowly to mix the juice with saliva. Don't gulp them down.

6. Peel oranges and grapefruits, but be sure and leave on the white, pithy part of the peel. That is the part that contains the important bioflavonoids. Leave the skins on all other organic fruits and vegetables. Remove the green top portion from carrots, since they may contain a toxic substance. Slice the fruits and vegetables so that they fit nicely into your juicer.

7. Drink the juices immediately after juicing—do not store them. As soon as a fruit or vegetable is sliced, it begins to lose nutritional value.

8. If you do not have time to juice fruits and vegetables, simply take one of the phytonutrient powders listed in Appendix B. These powders contain organic vegetables and fruits. Preparation is easy: simply mix with water and shake in a shaker cup or travel mug. In other words, you can prepare your juiced meal in twenty seconds or less. Remember to sip slowly.

9. Transfer your juice from the juicer to the blender and add crushed ice to create delicious smoothies from any juice recipe.

10. If your juicer spits out the fiber (pulp) from your fruits and veggies, which most juicers do, add 1 to 2 teaspoons of the fiber back into the juice before you drink it. The fiber helps to regulate your blood sugar, lowers cholesterol, prevents gallstones, and binds toxins.

BEST FRUIT AND VEGGIE CHOICES

When you are juicing, keep in mind that some fruits and vegetables provide more health benefits than others. Fruits and veggies that are especially cleansing on the juice fast include:

- Cabbage and other cruciferous vegetables
- Greens
- Dandelion root and dandelion greens
- Sprouts
- Celery
- Carrots
- Lemons and limes
- Apples
- Beets
- Berries (blueberries, blackberries, and strawberries)

For optimum detoxification, drink one juice drink a day that contains cruciferous vegetables such as cabbage, broccoli, or beets. The phytonutrients in these vegetables detoxify your body by helping to cleanse your liver and enhancing the flow of bile. You may want to include dandelion greens or dandelion root to support your liver in its detoxification efforts during the fast, too.

THE BASICS OF JUICE FASTING

In the next few pages you will find numerous delicious and healthful juicing combinations. *However, they are simply guides to help you find your own favorites.* Be creative! Make your own combinations and experiment with juicing.

When you create your own juices, there are four main fruits and vegetables that should usually form the base of each juice. These include carrots, celery, apples, and tomatoes. One of these, or a combination of them, should make up the greatest portion of your juice. You will find that they taste good and combine well with other fruits and vegetables. In addition, they are able to disguise the taste of veggies you may not like, such as cabbage and greens.

When you add organic greens, such as collard greens, spinach, broccoli, parsley, wheat grass or dandelion greens, they should make up no more than one-fourth of the juice. If you use more, you may not enjoy the taste. The recipes should make 8–12 ounces of juice, but some may make 16 ounces, depending on the size of your fruits and vegetables.

PHYSICAL RESPONSES TO THE FASTING PROGRAM

Your body may experience some interesting changes while fasting, so it is important to be aware of them before you begin. Not everyone will experience all of these physical responses, but in case you do, you need not be alarmed; just take necessary precautions if they occur. For example, you may experience:

- *Light-headedness.* This is a common physical response to fasting. To avoid this uncomfortable sensation, do not stand up quickly from a lying or sitting posture. If light-headedness does occur, lie down for a few minutes, and elevate your feet on some pillows.

- *Cold hands and feet.* It is common to experience a lowering of body temperature during a fast. The result can often be cold hands and feet. I suggest that you simply use an extra blanket at night and wear extra clothing for warmth.

- *Changes in energy.* While some people become fatigued during a fast, others actually feel more energetic. Either extreme should not alarm you. You may initially feel fatigued but gain new energy levels as your body begins to detoxify.

- *A change in sleep habits.* Your body may not require as much sleep as you are accustomed to requiring. Do not let this phenomenon alarm you. You need to plan to get plenty of rest during a fast, taking an afternoon siesta for about an hour if possible. I recommend that you limit strenuous exercise during the fast, taking leisurely strolls in a park or other slow, relaxing activities.

- *A coated tongue.* A very common symptom during fasting is the development of a white or yellow film on your tongue. This coating of the tongue signals a detoxification of your body.

- *Bad breath.* As toxins continue to be released from your body, your breath may take on an unpleasant odor. I suggest that you keep a toothbrush close at hand and that you brush your teeth and tongue often with organic toothpaste such as Tom's of Maine brand.

- *Constipation.* Especially during longer fasts, constipation can become a problem. To help prevent this problem, I recommend adding back 1 or 2 teaspoons of fiber with each juiced drink. Also, herbal teas can help to prevent constipation, as can using a scoop of phytonutrient powder in water or added to one of the daily juices you consume. (See Appendix B.)

- *Skin eruptions.* Toxins released through fasting may result in eruptions of boils, rashes, or acne as the body detoxifies using the largest excretory organ, the skin.

- *Body odor.* As toxins exit the body through the sweat glands, some individuals will develop a body odor. Warm baths help the skin and glands to slough off these toxins. Sauna and infrared sauna therapy is also effective. (See Appendix B.)

- *Darker than normal urine.* This indicates one of two things: either you are shedding large quantities of toxins through the urine, or you are not consuming adequate liquids. In either case, you need to increase your fluid intake.

- *Mucus drainage.* You may experience mucus drainage from your sinuses, bronchial tubes, or GI tract. Do not be alarmed. Again, these symptoms simply indicate that your body is using this system as well for voiding itself of many of the built-up toxins it has been storing.

- *Nausea and vomiting.* If you become mildly dehydrated, you may experience nausea and vomiting. Be sure to get enough fluids during your fast, especially the clean, pure water that is so important to cleansing your body. Please do not consume tap water.

SPECIAL PRECAUTIONS FOR SPECIAL HEALTH ISSUES

If your state of health is less than desirable at present, you may reap great benefits from fasting. However, you should also take special precautions to address your health issues before considering a fast. The following health issues require some attention to ensure that fasting will be beneficial, not harmful.

Candidiasis, food allergies, parasites

If you experience symptoms of excessive bloating, gas, and diarrhea, you may be suffering from candidiasis, bacterial overgrowth in the small intestines, or even a parasitic infection. These symptoms may also signal malabsorption, maldigestion, increased intestinal permeability, food allergies, or food sensitivities. If you have any of these symptoms, I strongly recommend that you get a comprehensive digestive stool analysis with parasitology, a test for intestinal permeability, and a food allergy test before you decide to fast. In addition, I recommend that you read my book *The Bible Cure for Candida and Yeast Infections* and follow the special diet it contains for three months before you start fasting.

Hypoglycemia

If you suffer from hypoglycemia, you may need to maintain a constant blood sugar level by drinking juice every two or three hours while fasting, instead of only four or five times a day. Also, I recommend that you add back 1 or 2 teaspoons of the pulp or fiber to each juiced drink you consume.

GI tract sensitivities

Some who suffer from sensitive GI tract symptoms, such as pain, bloating, gas, or diarrhea after drinking a certain kind of juice, simply need to omit that fruit or vegetable and try another one. By process of elimination, you will be able to identify the fruit of vegetable to which your GI tract is sensitive and then avoid using it during your fast. Also, some patients with sensitive GI tracts show less symptoms when they separate vegetable and fruit juices instead of drinking them in combination.

STARTING YOUR JUICE FASTING PROGRAM

If you are ready, the following pages will guide you day by day through your seven-day juice fast, complete with recipes and room for journaling your experience. I am convinced that you will be so satisfied with the improvement of your health that juice fasting brings that you will want to make juice fasting a regular part of your new fasted lifestyle.

JUICE FASTING
Days 22–28

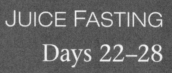

DR. COLBERT'S JUICE FAST DAY 22

MEAL SUGGESTIONS

Breakfast–Juice:	Snack–Juice:	Lunch–Juice:	Dinner–Juice:
½ small lemon or lime, peeled 1 cup berries 3 oranges, peeled 1 scoop phytonutrient powder (optional; see Appendix B)	2 celery stalks 2 apples, cored and seeded 2 carrots	1 beet 2 carrots 2 celery stalks ½ sweet potato, raw	4 medium tomatoes 2 celery stalks ½ cucumber Handful of bean or broccoli sprouts 1 clove garlic (optional)

FOCUS THOUGHT

The ancient father of medicine, Hippocrates, said, "Everything in excess is opposed by nature." Many years as a practicing medical doctor have convinced me that he was right.

YOUR DAILY PRESCRIPTION FOR HEALTH

Our nation is suffering an epidemic of degenerative diseases and death that is caused by excess—plain and simple. We have eaten too much sugar, too much fat, too much meat, too many empty calories, and far too much processed, devitalized food.

Detoxification through fasting can turn your life and health around. It is a natural, biblical system of supporting and cleansing the body from built-up chemicals, fats, and other toxins. Periodic fasting will allow you to eliminate and live free of the physical and neurological burden of toxins.

The juice fast phase of the twenty-eight-day fasting program may be the most difficult to complete, but it can offer you the greatest benefits. Find a verse from the Bible that you will use to encourage and inspire you during this important phase. Write it on the lines below:

_____

_____

_____

YOUR DAILY SPIRITUAL JOURNEY

Then Esther told them to reply to Mordecai: "Go, gather all the Jews who are present in Shushan, and fast for me; neither eat nor drink for three days, night or day. My maids and I will fast likewise. And so I will go to the king, which is against the law; and if I perish, I perish."

—ESTHER 4:15–16

Queen Esther understood the value of fasting in order to receive God's protection and His favor in tough situations. Faced with great danger to her people and herself, Queen Esther called a fast. (See Esther 4.) The three days of corporate fasting called by Esther turned the situation around completely in a mighty display of supernatural favor and power. Haman, who had plotted to annihilate the Jews, was exposed and hung from the very same gallows he had built to hang Esther's cousin Mordecai.

Fasting will provide you with protection, deliverance, and divine favor, and it reveals the power of fasting to move the hand of God mightily and to change the hearts of men. What circumstances do you need God's help with?

- ☐ Protection and deliverance from domestic violence
- ☐ Safety from physical harm
- ☐ Protection of your home, finances, and business
- ☐ For safety and protection of your children in school, day care, or any other public place

Let's declare God's protection and peace of mind. You can pray this prayer or a similar one in your own words.

Dear Lord, Your Word promises to keep me in perfect peace when my mind is stayed on You. I claim this peace for my life today as I trust You for Your safety and protection in my life and my family members' lives. In Jesus' name, amen.

RECORD YOUR THOUGHTS

Use the space provided to record what God is laying on your heart during your prayer time today.

_____

_____

_____

DAY 23 / DR. COLBERT'S JUICE FAST

MEAL SUGGESTIONS

Breakfast–Juice:	Snack–Juice:	Lunch–Juice:	Dinner–Juice:
1 pink grapefruit, peeled ½ small lemon or lime, peeled 1 apple, cored and seeded 1 scoop phytonutrient powder (optional; see Appendix B)	Cut watermelon in sections and remove seeds. Juice enough melon for 8–12 ounces of juice.	½ head cabbage Handful collard greens 2 carrots 1 apple, cored and seeded	2 carrots 1 beet ½ cucumber 2 celery stalks

FOCUS THOUGHT

Using the right kinds of raw, fresh juices increases the healing benefits of fasting.

YOUR DAILY PRESCRIPTION FOR HEALTH

Since fresh juices are very easy for the body to assimilate, they give your digestive tract a chance to rest and repair. Juice fasting also creates an alkaline environment for your body's cells and tissues so that they can start releasing waste products through your body's various channels of elimination. The primary elimination channels of the body include the kidneys and urinary tract, the colon, the lungs, and the skin. Fasting allows your liver to catch up on its internal cleansing and detoxification. At the same time, the digestive organs, including the stomach, pancreas, intestines, and gallbladder, get a much-deserved rest.

Even the blood and the lymphatic system can be effectively cleansed of toxic buildup through fasting. During fasting, our cells, tissues, and organs can begin to dump out accumulated waste products of cellular metabolism as well as chemicals and other toxins. This helps your cells to heal, repair, and be strengthened. You have about sixty to one hundred trillion cells in your body, and each one takes in nutrients and produces waste products. Fasting allows each cell to dump its waste products and thus be able to function at peak efficiency.

Fatty tissues release chemicals and toxins during fasting. These, in turn, are broken down by the liver, excreted by the kidneys and through the bile. Your body will excrete toxins in many different ways during fasting. Some people actually develop boils, rashes, or body odor during fasting since toxins are being released through the body's largest excretory organ, the skin.

YOUR DAILY SPIRITUAL JOURNEY

The Lord will guide you continually.

—ISAIAH 58:11

To realize all of the benefits of fasting, you must be led by the Spirit during this special time. Spend some time reading about fasting and about the Spirit of God in the Bible. Start with Luke 4, which explains how Jesus was led by the Spirit to fast in the desert for forty days. When He returned from His fast, He was full of power and full of the Spirit.

You should fast when a need or situation in life calls for it. If you have a great need to hear from the Lord, the Spirit will usually lead you into a fast. Write out a prayer of thanks to God for leading you to fast.

_____

_____

_____

Say your prayer aloud and repeat it as He answers your prayers, bringing the comfort and guidance you need.

RECORD YOUR THOUGHTS

Use the space provided to record any answers to prayer or guidance you feel the Lord is giving to you.

_____

_____

_____

_____

DR. COLBERT'S JUICE FAST | DAY 24

MEAL SUGGESTIONS

Breakfast–Juice:	Snack–Juice:	Lunch–Juice:	Dinner–Juice:
Handful of parsley 2 apples, cored and seeded 1 scoop phytonutrient powder (optional; see Appendix B)	3-inch slice pineapple with skin ¼ inch ginger root Handful of parsley	Handful of parsley 1 tomato 2 celery stalks 1 garlic clove (optional)	3 carrots Handful of collard greens, spinach, or beet greens 1 garlic clove Handful of parsley

FOCUS THOUGHT

You have it within your power to provide your incredible liver and GI tract with enough help so that they can once again function at peak efficiency.

YOUR DAILY PRESCRIPTION FOR HEALTH

A simple juice fast called the Lemonade Fast or the "Master Cleanse" has been around for quite a while, and tens of thousands have benefited from this powerful fast, which helps your body's natural ability to detoxify, keeping it from getting overloaded with environmental as well as dietary toxins. Use the following recipe for your "Master Cleanse."[5]

---

2 Tbsp. fresh squeezed lemon or lime juice
1 Tbsp. 100 percent pure maple syrup (from a health food store)
Dash of cayenne pepper
8 oz. pure, clean water
Liquid stevia to taste

Mix and drink eight to twelve glasses a day. For more information, refer to my book *Toxic Relief.*

YOUR DAILY SPIRITUAL JOURNEY

Is it not to share your bread with the hungry, and that you bring to your house the poor who are cast out?... The Lord will guide you continually, and satisfy your soul in drought, and strengthen your bones.

—ISAIAH 58:7, 11

It may come as a shock to some, but just as fasting breaks the grip of toxins and brings the blessing of health to your body, I believe that fasting breaks poverty and releases the blessings of prosperity in your life. If you plant a seed through giving as you fast, I believe a major blessing will return to you quickly. Now, this doesn't necessarily mean that you will become rich, but God's power can break the cycle of poverty that tries to prevent you from giving to God's work and helping others in their time of need. In the quote from Isaiah 58, the fasting chapter, we see that God promises to satisfy us in times of drought. Perhaps circumstances in your life right now are creating a financial drought. God is able to provide what you need so that you, in turn, can be a blessing to someone else. Describe a financial situation that you want to see God turn around for you or someone you know during this time of fasting.

_____

_____

_____

Dear Lord, I believe Your Word applies to my life, and I claim it for my financial situation. I believe that as I humble myself before You by fasting and as I obey Your Word by giving my tithes and offerings, You will honor my obedience with a thirty-, sixty-, or even a hundredfold blessing. I thank You in advance for the blessing and provision You are about to bring forth in my life. In Jesus' name, amen.

RECORD YOUR THOUGHTS

Use the space provided to record what you sense the Lord is laying on your heart as you pray today.

_____

_____

_____

_____

DR. COLBERT'S JUICE FAST · DAY 25

MEAL SUGGESTIONS

Breakfast–Juice:	Snack–Juice:	Lunch–Juice:	Dinner–Juice:
2 celery stalks 2 apples, cored and seeded 2 carrots 1 scoop phytonutrient powder (optional; see Appendix B)	1 large cucumber 3 stalks celery 2 large carrots 1 bell pepper ¼ head green cabbage ½ bunch parsley	3 large tomatoes ½ bunch cilantro 1 fresh mild jalapeno 1 sweet red pepper 2 stalks celery ½ sweet onion	1 small beet (peeled) 3 large carrots ½ bunch parsley 2 stalks celery ¼ head cabbage 1 apple

FOCUS THOUGHT

The power of better health through detoxification is yours. Pursue your own good health aggressively by looking carefully at your diet and lifestyle. Your healthy future is in your hands.

YOUR DAILY PRESCRIPTION FOR HEALTH

The sensible, medically sound method of juice fasting can very quickly allow you to shed any extra toxic fat that your body may be carrying—even if you are significantly overweight. In addition, you can avoid a water-only fasting trap of which many people are not even aware. What's the trap? Water-only fasting can actually cause you to gain significant amounts of weight after the fast! That's one of the reasons that fasting with a program of specially prepared juices is so much more sensible. Not only that, but it's also much easier to stay on a specially prepared juice fast because your body will not crave nutrition in the same way that it does during a water-only fast.

YOUR DAILY SPIRITUAL JOURNEY

When they were sick, my clothing was sackcloth; I humbled myself with fasting.

—PSALM 35:13

What does it mean to overcome the flesh? In simple terms, it means to humble or discipline yourself. In Psalm 69:10, David writes that fasting "chastened" his soul. Chastening is a type of discipline that refines and purifies. It's a time of pruning back the dead areas of your life so that God can renew His life and purpose within you. What are some areas where you have been lacking discipline that you now sense God leading you to prune away?

_____

_____

_____

Is weight control or weight loss one of the benefits you want to achieve? What factors do you believe have contributed to your being overweight? What amount of weight do you think you need to lose to reach your optimal health?

_____

_____

_____

As you near the completion of this physical fast, think about other areas of your life where you could benefit through a "fast." Are there emotions and feelings that you would like to eliminate from your life (fear, anger, anxiety, unforgiveness, depression, grief, guilt, shame, and so forth)? What habits or actions keep you from total health—body, mind, and spirit? List these below:

_____

_____

_____

Dear Lord, I thank You for giving me the power to have victory over my flesh as I continue with my fast. I pray that You will show me other areas of my life that may need to be "fasted" or abstained from so that I might achieve total health in my mind, body, and spirit. In Jesus' name, amen.

RECORD YOUR THOUGHTS

Use the space provided to record what you sense God is laying on your heart during your prayer time today.

_____

_____

_____

DAY 26

DR. COLBERT'S JUICE FAST

MEAL SUGGESTIONS

Breakfast–Juice:	Snack–Juice:	Lunch–Juice:	Dinner–Juice:
Cut watermelon in sections and remove seeds. Juice enough melon for 8–12 ounces of juice. Add 1 scoop phytonutrient powder (optional; see Appendix B).	1 cucumber 1 bell pepper 3 stalks celery ½ bunch parsley ¼ head cabbage 1 green apple	½ pineapple (peeled) 1 apple 2 carrots 1 small beet (peeled) 1 cup broccoli	1 cup broccoli ½ bunch parsley 2 stalks celery 1 cucumber ¼ head cabbage 1 bell pepper 1 lemon

FOCUS THOUGHT

When you get into the habit of juicing fruit and vegetables or consuming phytonutrient powders, you will dramatically reduce your risk of heart disease, cancer, stroke, diabetes, osteoporosis, macular degeneration, and all degenerative diseases.

YOUR DAILY PRESCRIPTION FOR HEALTH

The USDA, the Surgeon General, and the National Cancer Institute, as well as the U.S. Department of Health and Human Services, all recommend that we eat plenty of fruits and vegetables. In fact, the USDA advises that we eat five to thirteen servings of fruits and vegetables a day in order to maintain health.[6] While some studies show that Americans are beginning to consume more vegetables, keep in mind that white potatoes account for 30 percent of the vegetables consumed by Americans, and one third of these potatoes are french fries.[7] Because we eat so little fruit and vegetables, many Americans suffer from nutritional deficiencies, including vitamin and mineral deficiencies.

To make matters worse, many studies show how depleted soil has affected the mineral content of vegetables and fruits. One observer compared the data from the USDA handbook from 1972 to the USDA food tables of today and found dramatic reductions in nutrient content. For example, nearly half the calcium and vitamin A in broccoli have disappeared. The vitamin A content in collard greens has fallen to nearly half its previous levels. Potassium dropped from 400 mg to 170 mg, and magnesium fell from 57 mg to only 9 mg. Cauliflower lost almost half of its vitamin C along with its thiamine and riboflavin. The calcium in pineapple went from 17 mg to 7 mg. Those astonishing losses in nutrients eventually will have a significant impact on your health.[8]

YOUR DAILY SPIRITUAL JOURNEY

But I discipline my body and bring it into subjection, lest, when I have preached to others, I myself should become disqualified.

—1 CORINTHIANS 9:27

Fasting builds character and integrity. It helps to overcome temptation and allows us to be led by the Spirit and, therefore, to walk in integrity. Fasting is not an end in itself. It is intended to cultivate a greater closeness to God and to create more of His character within us. Then we can become clearer channels of His Spirit and develop godliness in all of our relationships. List the areas of temptation you are gaining power to overcome as you continue your fast.

_____

_____

_____

Dear Lord, I thank You for using this time of fasting to create more of Your character in my life. My sole desire is to become like You and be used by You. Take complete control and have Your way in my life. Complete the character-building process You have begun during this fast. In Jesus' name, amen.

RECORD YOUR THOUGHTS

Use the space provided to record what you sense God is laying on your heart during your prayer time today.

_____

_____

_____

_____

DR. COLBERT'S JUICE FAST DAY 27

MEAL SUGGESTIONS

Breakfast–Juice:	Snack–Juice:	Lunch–Juice:	Dinner–Juice:
3-inch slice pineapple with skin ¼ inch ginger root Handful of parsley 1 scoop phytonutrient powder (optional; see Appendix B)	2 oranges 1 lemon 1 grapefruit 2 tangerines 2 carrots 2 stalks celery	2 garlic cloves ½ cucumber 2 celery stalks Handful of spinach	2 tomatoes 1 cucumber 2 celery stalks 1 garlic clove

FOCUS THOUGHT

Determine to make juicing fresh fruits and vegetables a part of your daily breakfast routine in your new health-first lifestyle.

YOUR DAILY PRESCRIPTION FOR HEALTH

Many believe that they can fast one time and go back to eating the same high-fat, high-sugar, high-processed starches, and high-meat diet that caused them to develop the degenerative diseases in the first place. That would be the same as saying that if a person stopped smoking for a month, then he could go back and start smoking his two packs of cigarettes a day. Don't go back to the old unhealthy habits. Instead, let your detoxification program and fast be the beginning of a new, healthier lifestyle.

And speaking of smoking, every time a smoker puffs on a cigarette or cigar he plants a seed for lung cancer and heart disease. How true the Bible is when it warns that the seeds we sow are the plants we will reap. (See Galatians 6:7.) If you continue to smoke, you will eventually harvest disease. So, stop smoking and start juicing. Juicing is one of the best ways to break an addiction to cigarettes—and other addictions as well.

YOUR DAILY SPIRITUAL JOURNEY

Most assuredly, I say to you, he who believes in Me, the works that I do he will do also; and greater works than these he will do, because I go to My Father. And whatever you ask in My name, that I will do, that the Father may be glorified in the Son. If you ask anything in My name, I will do it.

—JOHN 14:12–14

Jesus didn't begin His earthly ministry until He had fasted for forty days. The Holy Spirit led Him into the desert, and after His fast, He returned in the power of the Holy Spirit. This was when His mighty ministry was launched, a ministry of great miracles, signs, and wonders. All of this took place as a result of fasting.

Interestingly, Jesus told us that we too would do these works and even greater works because He went to the Father. I truly believe that we will see these greater works as we learn and practice the great spiritual discipline of fasting.

If Jesus Christ felt the need to fast, how much more should we? Describe the ministry you feel God is using this time of fasting to prepare you to do.

_____

_____

_____

Dear Lord, I believe You are equipping me to do Your work and be a minister of Your love and life to a dying world. Guide my feet, my hands, my thoughts, and my words as I set out to accomplish Your calling on my life. I thank You that You have promised to do anything that I ask in Your name. Amen.

RECORD YOUR THOUGHTS

Use the space provided to record what you sense God is laying on your heart during your prayer time today.

_____

_____

_____

_____

DAY 28

DR. COLBERT'S JUICE FAST

MEAL SUGGESTIONS

Breakfast–Juice:	Snack–Juice:	Lunch–Juice:	Dinner–Juice:
2 celery stalks 2 apples, cored and seeded 2 carrots 1 scoop phytonutrient powder (optional; see Appendix B)	½ head cabbage 2 celery stalks 2 carrots Handful of parsley	1 beet 2 carrots 2 celery stalks ½ sweet potato, raw	4 medium tomatoes 2 celery stalks ½ cucumber Handful of bean or broccoli sprouts 1 clove garlic (optional)

FOCUS THOUGHT

Hopefully, after this twenty-eight-day experience you will feel motivated to cleanse and detoxify your body on a regular basis and to establish a consistent health-first lifestyle for you and your family. For more information on choosing the healthiest foods, please refer to my books What Would Jesus Eat?[9] *and* The Seven Pillars of Health.

YOUR DAILY PRESCRIPTION FOR HEALTH

You have now completed the Dr. Colbert twenty-eight-day detox and cleansing fast. Spend some time reflecting on the experience. Look back through the things you've recorded in your journal, and write a brief summary of your experience. Were your goals reached? Did God have different goals that He revealed to you along the way? How do you feel different in mind, body, and spirit than you did twenty-eight days ago?

YOUR DAILY SPIRITUAL JOURNEY

And the vessel that he made of clay was marred in the hand of the potter; so he made it again into another vessel, as it seemed good to the potter to make.

—JEREMIAH 18:4

As you have journeyed through this twenty-eight-day fast, you have allowed God, the Master Potter, to complete His divine process of deconstruction and rebuilding in your life. Be encouraged that you are now a vessel that "seemed good to the potter to make." Of course, He will never be finished working on any of us, but every time we submit ourselves to Him, we ask Him to reshape and remold us into His likeness, and we are refined and purified. Spend a moment in prayer, thanking God for His refining process in your life.

Dear Lord, I thank You that You love and accept me as I am, but that You are ever refashioning and reshaping my life to make me a clearer reflection of You. As I end this time of fasting and return to some of my regular daily routines, I ask for wisdom and protection from enemy attacks. Thank You, Lord, for leading me and loving me. In Jesus' name, amen.

RECORD YOUR THOUGHTS

Use the space provided to record what you sense God is laying on your heart during your prayer time today.

_____

_____

_____

CHAPTER 9

Breaking My Fast

You have come to the very important phase of breaking your fast. This is often the most difficult and most important part of fasting. Therefore, you must understand how to break your fast before you even begin.

Reintroduce foods gradually to realize the greatest health benefits of fasting. Your digestive tract has been at rest. That means hydrochloric acid and pancreatic enzymes may not be available to help you digest proteins, starches, and fats right away. Therefore, the longer your fast time, the more slowly you should come off of your fast.

Some individuals who have not broken their fast properly have developed gallstones and have needed surgery. I gradually reintroduce fruit, then vegetables, then starches such as breads, and finally proteins and fats. Some may find it beneficial to take 1–2 tablespoons of lecithin granules (in 2 ounces of water) once or twice daily to prevent sludge in the gallbladder during this stage of the program.

Follow this four-day phase of breaking your fast to insure the good health you have begun to achieve through the first two phases of my fasting program. If this was your first experience with a detoxifying fast, or if you suffer from poor health or numerous diseases, at the end of the four days you may repeat the twenty-one-day liver support phase of my fasting program before you move on to a healthy lifestyle described in my book *What Would Jesus Eat?*

Your journey to good health is not over when the next four days have ended. Your journey is just beginning. Be ready to step into your new health-first lifestyle plan with these first four days after your fast.

THE FIRST DAY AFTER YOUR FAST

The first day after your fast, eat fresh fruit such as apples, watermelon, grapes, or fresh berries as often as every two to three hours on the first day that your fast is broken. However, don't eat papaya or pineapple on the first day after a fast. These fruits contain strong enzymes that may upset your stomach. Fruits with the highest water content, such as watermelon, are the easiest to digest.

Have you prepared your shopping list to begin your new health-first lifestyle? Begin your shopping list today. When you go to the grocery store, shop for the following organic fruits and vegetables: carrots, cabbage, apples, cucumbers, beets, celery, parsley, berries (including strawberries, blackberries, blueberries, raspberries), lemons and limes, grapefruit, pineapple, ginger root, watermelon, garlic, greens (including spinach, collard greens, beet greens, dandelion greens), tomatoes, sweet potatoes, and dandelion root.

Juice or meal suggestions

Breakfast

- 1 cup sliced strawberries
- 1 scoop phytonutrient powder (optional; see Appendix B)

Snack drink

- 2 celery stalks
- 2 apples
- 2 carrots

Lunch

- ½ cup each: grapes, mixed berries, apple slices

Evening meal

- 1 cup watermelon chunks
- 1 cup grapes
- 1 small apple, sliced or chunks

Snack

- Fresh or frozen grapes

Daily supplements

- A multivitamin daily (see Appendix B)
- A scoop of phytonutrient powder (see Appendix B)

THE SECOND DAY AFTER YOUR FAST

On the second day after the fast is broken, have fruit in the morning. For lunch and dinner, have a bowl of fresh vegetable soup. Avoid creamy soups. Eat slowly and chew your food very well. Be sure not to overeat. Be sure you continue to drink at least two quarts of clean, pure water a day. You may also continue to drink your juices once or twice a day.

Juice or meal suggestions

Breakfast

- 1 cup mixed berries
- ½ cup grapes
- 1 scoop phytonutrient powder (optional: see Appendix B)

Snack drink

- A handful of parsley
- 4 carrots
- 1 apple

Lunch

- 1 bowl fresh vegetable soup

Evening meal

- 1 bowl fresh vegetable soup

THE THIRD DAY AFTER YOUR FAST

On the third day, you may add to the fruit and vegetable soup a salad and/or a baked potato. You may also add a slice of whole-grain bread such as Ezekiel or manna bread, brown rice bread, or millet bread.

Juice or meal suggestions

Breakfast

- Sliced apples or applesauce on 1 slice toasted Ezekiel, millet, or brown rice bread
- ½ cup mixed berries
- 1 scoop phytonutrient powder (optional; see Appendix B)

Snack

- Carrot and celery sticks

Lunch

- Bowl of fresh vegetable soup
- Small vegetable salad

Dinner

- Baked potato
- Fresh vegetable soup
- 1 slice millet bread

THE FOURTH DAY AFTER YOUR FAST

On the fourth day, you may introduce a small amount (1 or 2 ounces) of free-range or organic chicken, turkey, fish, or lean meat. I recommend that you try one of the following healthy methods for preparing your foods.

- Lightly steaming your vegetables causes very little loss of nutrients.

- Stir-frying is a good method of cooking because the food is briefly cooked so that it retains most of its nutrients.

- Grilling is an acceptable means of food preparation. When grilling your free-range or organic meats, simply avoid charring the meat.

Juice or meal suggestions

Breakfast

- 1 small glass fruit juice
- 1 cup oatmeal mixed with ½ cup strawberries
- 1 scoop phytonutrient powder (optional; see Appendix B)

Snack

- Sliced apple with fresh grapes

Lunch

- Fresh vegetable salad
- 1–2 oz. grilled chicken breast

Dinner

- 1 cup fresh vegetable soup
- Small vegetable salad
- 1–2 oz. chicken, fish, or turkey
- Baked potato with one pat of organic butter

CONCLUSION

I trust that you have discovered that fasting is a powerful tool for health, cleansing, corporate strength, and spiritual empowerment. The Bible gives fasting an ancient position of honor, a place beside other dynamic principles for health and spiritual growth.

Fasting is a privilege, and it is a biblical key to cleansing that will bless your life with the gift of health, healing, renewed vitality, longevity, and deeper spirituality.

In this twenty-eight-day fasting program we have addressed comprehensively the wonderful benefits of cleansing the body through fasting. And I have helped you to understand the physical and spiritual benefits of living a fasted lifestyle.

I recommend that you choose to fast periodically for detoxification purposes and that you commit your fasting time to God for spiritual cleansing and renewal as well. I commend you for your diligence during my twenty-eight-day fasting program and for the courage to establish a new health-first lifestyle plan for continued good health for you and your family.

As you begin to undergo periodic juice fasts for detoxification, I encourage you to first commit that time to God for spiritual cleansing and renewal. Once you become accustomed to fasting for two or three days, you may choose to increase that time a little. Learn to devote increasing portions of that time to Bible reading, prayer, and journaling for personal and spiritual growth. At times you may even choose to commit your fast times to even higher purposes, such as fasting for issues of national cleansing and healing.

As you develop a health-first lifestyle of fasting and prayer, you will walk in the footsteps of great men and women who have gone before us—men and women who increased in purity of body, mind, and spirit, and who touched heaven with their prayers and nations with their passion.

APPENDIX A

Recipes for Weeks 1–3

As you are preparing the recipes in this section, here are some general guidelines: Use all organic ingredients, and use all fresh ingredients unless otherwise indicated. If canned foods are indicated, read labels carefully. Always use non-irradiated spices.

All recipes marked with an asterisk (*) appear courtesy of Ed and Elisa McClure, founders of the ZOE 8 Weight Management Program and authors of *Eat Your Way to a Healthy Life.*

BREAKFAST RECIPES

EASY BREAKFAST WRAPS
4 medium Ezekiel tortillas
2 tsp. almond butter
2 cups diced peaches
2 cups diced pears
Cinnamon to taste
Agave nectar (optional)

Warm the tortillas in the oven; then spread almond butter on each tortilla. Add peaches, pears, and cinnamon. Drizzle with agave if added sweetness is desired. Fold in the ends of the tortillas, roll tightly, and place in heated skillet, cooking until all sides are lightly browned. *Serves 4.*

. . . .

TIP: *Substitute peaches and pears with apples, bananas, or your favorite fresh fruit.*

CINNAMON OATS

1 cup steel-cut or rolled oats
1 tsp. agave nectar
½ cup dried currants
Stevia to taste (optional)
1⅓ cup clean, pure water
¼ cup crushed pineapple
1 tsp. cinnamon
1 tsp. nutmeg

Boil oats, agave, currants, and stevia in clean, pure water. Reduce heat and add remaining ingredients. Cook for 15–20 minutes, stirring occasionally. Serve hot. **Serves 1.**

TIP: *Stevia is a natural herb sweetener that comes in both powder and liquid form. When adding stevia to increase sweetness, do not add more than 1/16 tsp. at a time.*

MUESLI*

2 cups steel-cut or rolled oats
¼ cup pecans, chopped
¼ cup almonds
¼ cup walnuts
¼ cup sunflower seeds
¼ cup organic raisins
¼ cup dried currants

Mix all ingredients thoroughly and store in an airtight glass container. No cooking involved! To serve, moisten with coconut milk. **Serves 2.**

TIP: *Substitute fresh berries or halved grapes for raisins and currants.*

TEX-MEX BAGELS

2 Ezekiel bagels
Quick Guacamole (page 186)
1 medium red onion, sliced
2 stalks green onion, chopped
1 tomato, sliced
1 avocado, sliced
2 Tbsp. sprouts

Split bagels and toast in toaster oven. Spread bagel slices with guacamole. Top with onions, tomato, avocado, and sprouts. ***Serves 4***.

TIP: *Spread two bagel halves with refried black beans instead of guacamole, or serve beans on the side.*

BUCKWHEAT PANCAKES

(Adapted from *The Peaceful Palate* by Jennifer Raymond)

1 cup buckwheat flour

1 tsp. active dry yeast

Pinch of sea salt

1½ cups warm water

¼ tsp. baking soda

1 tsp. molasses

1 cup fresh blueberries

Preheat oven to 200 degrees. Mix flour, yeast, and salt in large bowl. Add 1¼ cups warm water and beat until very smooth. Place in oven and turn the oven off. Allow dough to rise in the oven until bubbly, about 1 hour. Dissolve soda and molasses in ¼ cup warm water and add to buckwheat batter. Mix well, then let stand 30 minutes.

Lightly spray or brush skillet with olive oil. When heated, pour small amounts of batter and cook until bubbly. Flip and cook second side about 1 minute. Top with blueberries and serve. ***Makes about 10 3-inch pancakes***.

BROWN RICE GRITS*

¼ cup Arrowhead Mills Rise & Shine cereal

¾ cup clean, pure water

¼ cup unsweetened coconut milk

1 tsp. pecans, chopped

¼ tsp. cinnamon

Stevia to taste (optional)

Add cereal to clean, pure water and bring to boil, stirring constantly. Reduce heat, cover, and simmer for about 2 minutes, until desired consistency is reached. Place in serving bowls; add remaining ingredients as desired to enhance flavor. ***Serves 1***.

BREAKFAST SWEET POTATOES

2 cups sweet potatoes, peeled and cubed

½ cup rice or almond milk

Agave nectar (optional)
Cinnamon (optional)

Place sweet potatoes in pot and mash them, adding milk until they reach the consistency of Cream of Wheat cereal. Cook over medium heat until warmed through, stirring occasionally. Add agave and cinnamon to taste, if desired. **Serves 2**.

TOASTED BAGEL

2 Ezekiel bagels
2 Tbsp. almond butter
1 cup red or white grapes, halved

Split bagels and toast. Spread with almond butter and top with grapes. **Serves 2**.

HOT AND CREAMY CEREAL*

⅔ cup quinoa flakes
⅓ cup rice or almond milk
1 tsp. pecans, chopped
Stevia to taste (optional)

Prepare flakes according to package directions. Moisten with milk. Top with pecans and stevia, if desired. **Serves 1**.

TIP: *You can substitute steel-cut or rolled oats for quinoa flakes.*

BREAKFAST TACOS

1 Tbsp. extra-virgin olive oil
½ onion, chopped
½ capsicum, chopped
1 clove garlic, crushed
2 cups tomato, diced (separate ½ cup after dicing)
2 Tbsp. tomato paste
¼ tsp. cumin
¼ tsp. coriander
¼ tsp. crushed red pepper
1 cup kidney or pinto beans
6 spelt taco shells
4 oz. romaine lettuce, shredded

Soak beans overnight (8 hours) in 6 to 8 cups of clean, pure water. Drain water and set beans aside.

Heat olive oil in medium skillet and sauté onion, capsicum, and garlic until translucent. Add 1½ cups of diced tomatoes, tomato paste, cumin, coriander, and crushed red pepper. Simmer for 10 minutes, adding beans halfway through simmering time. Heat taco shells according to package directions. Spoon bean filling into shells and top with remaining tomatoes and lettuce. **Serves 4.**

TIP: *For a lighter taste, sauté in vegetable broth instead of olive oil.*

PECAN QUINOA*

½ cup uncooked quinoa
1½ tsp. extra-virgin olive oil
¼ tsp. garlic, chopped
1 cup vegetable broth
1 Tbsp. pecans, chopped
1 tsp. fresh parsley, chopped
⅛ tsp. white pepper
Sea salt to taste

Rinse and drain quinoa thoroughly. In a 1½ quart saucepan, heat olive oil and lightly sauté garlic. Add quinoa, broth, pecans, parsley, pepper, and salt; bring to a boil. Reduce heat and simmer until all water is absorbed (10–15 min). Mix and serve. **Serves 4.**

TIP: *You can substitute brown rice for quinoa. Prepare rice according to package instructions and follow remaining directions above.*

BANANA NUT CEREAL

1 cup steel-cut or rolled oats
¼ cup quinoa flakes
Clean, pure water
¼ pecans, chopped
2 Tbsp. agave nectar
1 banana, mashed
Cinnamon to taste

Mix oats and quinoa. Cook in enough clean, pure water to obtain consistency of Cream of Wheat cereal. Add remaining ingredients. **Serves 2.**

EGG-LESS FRENCH TOAST

1 cup rice or almond milk
3 Tbsp. arrowroot powder
1 tsp. orange juice concentrate
1 tsp. agave nectar
1 tsp. vanilla
Pinch of sea salt
4 slices millet bread
Cinnamon to taste (optional)
2 cups fresh fruit of your choice

Combine milk, arrowroot, orange juice, agave, vanilla, and salt in baking dish until thoroughly mixed. Dip bread into mixture, one slice at a time, until both sides are evenly coated. Lightly spray or brush skillet with olive oil and brown soaked bread over medium heat until both sides are golden (about 3 minutes per side). Place on serving plate and drizzle with agave. Sprinkle with cinnamon if desired, and top with fresh fruit. **Serves 2.**

OATMEAL WAFFLES

(Adapted from **The Peaceful Palate** *by Jennifer Raymond)*
1 cup rolled oats
1 cup clean, pure water
½ banana
2 tsp. agave nectar
½ tsp. vanilla
Sea salt to taste

Blend all ingredients on high speed until smooth. If batter is too thick to pour, add more water until pancake batter consistency is achieved. Lightly spray or brush heated waffle iron with olive oil before pouring batter into it. Cook according to waffle iron directions (about 10 minutes). Serve with agave nectar (instead of syrup) and fresh fruit. **Makes 4 waffles.**

CRISPY BROWN RICE FLAKES

1 cup crispy brown rice flakes
½ cup rice or almond milk
Stevia to taste (optional)

Pour flakes into a bowl and moisten with milk. Sprinkle with very small amount of stevia powder if added sweetness is desired. **Serves 1.**

TIP: *Top with sliced banana or strawberries for added flavor.*

GREEN APPLE COMPOTE*

4 cups apples, chopped (peeled, if you prefer)
2 Tbsp. agave nectar
1 tsp. nutmeg
1 tsp. cinnamon
½ cup clean, pure water

Combine all ingredients in saucepan and simmer over medium-low heat, covered, until apples are soft (approximately 20 minutes). Cool and serve with Oatmeal Waffles (page 148). Refrigerate in airtight glass container for up to 3 days. ***Makes 3½ cups.***

TIP: *Substitute stevia for agave to reduce sugar grams and reach desired sweetness.*

FRESH BERRIES WITH LEMON-COCONUT SAUCE

1¾ cups coconut milk
2 Tbsp. lemon juice
¼ tsp. vanilla extract (check label; make sure no corn syrup added)
2 tsp. lemon zest
⅛ tsp. stevia (optional)
1½ tsp. arrowroot
¼ cup clean, pure water
4 cups of your favorite berry varieties

In small saucepan, mix milk, lemon juice, vanilla extract, and lemon zest. Bring to a boil. Reduce heat and simmer for 5 minutes, adding stevia if added sweetness is desired. Mix arrowroot and water. Add to lemon mixture and simmer until mixture is thick and creamy. Place berries in serving bowls and drizzle with sauce. Serve with a sprouted English muffin. ***Serves 8.***

CANTALOUPE-BERRY DELIGHT

1 cantaloupe, seeded and sliced
1 cup fresh berries (choose 2–3 of your favorite varieties)

Arrange cantaloupe slices on 2 plates. Spoon berries in heap in center of each plate. Serve with a spelt bagel. ***Serves 2.***

GINGER FRUIT MIX

1 lime (for juice)
1 Tbsp. ginger, minced
1 Tbsp. mint, minced
3 kiwis, chopped
2 oranges, chopped
2 peaches, chopped
2 apples, chopped
1 grapefruit, chopped
1 mango, chopped
½ pineapple, chopped
6 mint leaves

In small bowl, squeeze juice from lime. Add ginger and mint. Set aside. Combine all fruit in airtight glass container and toss with lime juice until evenly coated. Refrigerate for at least 15 minutes, tossing occasionally. Garnish with mint leaves and serve with toasted millet bread. ***Serves 6***.

FRESH FRUIT CUP

1 peach, peeled and diced
1 pear, peeled and diced
½ cup strawberries, halved with stems removed
½ cup cantaloupe, seeded and diced
½ cup blueberries
½ cup red or white grapes, halved
2 Tbsp. agave nectar (optional)

Combine fruit and agave. Stir until well mixed and fruit is evenly coated with agave. Serve in small bowls or cups along with two slices of Ezekiel bread. ***Serves 2***.

MIXED BERRY COMPOTE*

1 cup frozen unsweetened blueberries
1 cup frozen unsweetened strawberries
1 cup frozen unsweetened blackberries
1 cup clean, pure water
Stevia to taste
2 tsp. arrowroot powder

Place berries and 3/4 cup water in a small saucepan; cook about 15 minutes. Sweeten with stevia to taste. Mix ¼ cup water with arrowroot powder and add to mixture; simmer until thickened. Remove from heat. **Makes 3 cups.** Serve as a topping on Buckwheat Pancakes (page 145).

BAKED APPLES

2 golden apples
Clean, pure water
Cinnamon
2 sprouted tortillas (optional)

Core, peel, and slice apples. Cover surface of saucepan with water and warm over medium heat. Add apples to water. Sprinkle with cinnamon to taste. Simmer until apples are warmed through (about 5 minutes), stirring halfway through cook time. **Serves 2.**

TIP: *To feel fuller, try spooning the baked apple mixture onto sprouted tortillas and wrapping them burrito-style.*

SNACK RECIPES

SPICY SUNFLOWER SEEDS
(Requires advance preparation)

1 cup hulled sunflower seeds
¼ cup sesame seeds
1 Tbsp. Cajun Spice Mix (page 186)

Preheat oven to 350 degrees. Lightly spray or brush olive oil on a baking sheet. Place seeds on baking sheet; spray or brush lightly with olive oil. Sprinkle spice mix to lightly coat. Roast in oven until lightly browned, approximately 15 minutes; turn halfway through cooking process. Remove from oven. Toss and season once more, then let cool completely. Refrigerate in airtight glass container. **Makes 1¼ cups.**

GRANOLA CRUMBLE

3 cups steel-cut or rolled oats
1 cup hulled sunflower seeds (or nuts)
⅓ cup extra-virgin olive oil
2 bananas, extra ripe
1 Tbsp. agave nectar
1 medium apple, chopped

Preheat oven to 350 degrees. Mix oats, sunflower seeds, and olive oil. Set aside. Mash bananas and stir in agave nectar and apple. Add oat mixture, stirring well. Let sit for 30 minutes. Crumble mixture onto ungreased baking sheet and bake in oven for 15 minutes. Cool completely on baking sheet. Store in airtight glass container. ***Makes 5 cups.***

SPICY CHICKPEAS

4 Tbsp. extra-virgin olive oil
1 Tbsp. Cajun Spice Mix (page 186)
1 Tbsp. chili powder
1 tsp. sea salt
½ tsp. fresh ground pepper
15-oz. can chickpeas, drained and rinsed

Preheat oven to 400 degrees. In baking pan, mix oil and spices. Add chickpeas and stir until thoroughly coated. Bake in oven for 15–20 minutes, stirring halfway through bake time. Cool completely on baking dish. Store in airtight glass container. ***Makes 2 cups.***

TIP: *Canned beans are convenient, but it's better to purchase dried beans whenever possible. Soak 1 cup of beans overnight (approximately 8 hours) in 6 to 8 cups clean, pure water. Drain water and follow remaining directions.*

ASPARAGUS TAPENADE*

1 pound asparagus spears
1½ Tbsp. garlic, chopped
½ cup fresh basil
¼ cup pine nuts
½ tsp. sea salt
¼ tsp. fresh ground black pepper
3 Tbsp. extra-virgin olive oil

Peel and trim asparagus, then steam until tender but crisp (approximately 4–5 minutes). Chop asparagus and place in food processor; add remaining ingredients, except oil, and process. While processing, add the olive oil and continue processing until a paste consistency is reached. Spread on brown rice crackers. ***Serves 6.***

TIP: *Can also be served as a condiment or tossed with hot pasta.*

CAJUN NUT MIX*
(Use roasted nuts and seeds with no oil or salt added)
1 cup raw hulled sunflower seeds

1 cup pine nuts
1 cup pecan halves
1 cup pumpkin seeds
1 cup almonds
1 Tbsp. Cajun Spice Mix (page 186)
Sea salt

Preheat oven to 350 degrees. Lightly spray or brush olive oil on a baking sheet. Place nuts and seeds on baking sheet; spray or brush lightly with olive oil. Sprinkle Cajun Spice Mix and salt to lightly coat mixture. Roast mixture in oven until lightly browned, approximately 15 minutes; turn halfway through cooking process. Remove from oven. Toss and season once more, then let cool completely. Refrigerate in airtight glass container. **Makes 5 cups.**

ROASTED RED PEPPER WRAPS

1 red bell pepper, seeded and diced
1 small onion, diced
2 Tbsp. extra-virgin olive oil
Hummus (page 154)
2 Ezekiel tortillas
1 cup mixed salad greens

Sauté pepper and onion in olive oil until pepper skins begin to char. Remove from heat and allow to cool. Spread Hummus over tortillas. Be sure to spread evenly to the edges of the bread. When veggies are cool, spread over Hummus, leaving a 2-inch border of bread and Hummus so the wrap will "stick." Add salad greens. Tightly roll the wrap and refrigerate for 1 hour before serving. Do not refrigerate more than 1 hour, or bread will become soggy. **Serves 2.**

TIP: *Use toothpicks to hold wrap together, if needed.*

BANANA-ALMOND DELIGHT

1 banana, sliced
½ cup coconut milk
¼ cup almonds, chopped
Agave nectar (optional)

Place chopped banana in bowl. Pour milk over banana. Top with nuts and agave (if added sweetness is desired). **Serves 1.**

HUMMUS*

15-oz. can chickpeas (garbanzo beans), drained
2 Tbsp. extra-virgin olive oil
1 Tbsp. sesame oil
¼ tsp. cracked black pepper
1 tsp. fresh garlic
2 Tbsp. clean, pure water

Mix all ingredients in a small food processor until smooth. Serve with Belgian endive or brown rice crackers. **Serves 8**.

TIP: *Canned beans are convenient, but it's better to purchase dried beans whenever possible. Soak 1 cup of beans overnight (approximately 8 hours) in 6 to 8 cups clean, pure water. Drain water and follow remaining directions.*

BLACK BEAN DIP*

15-oz. can black beans, drained and rinsed
2 medium tomatoes, chopped
½ cup cilantro, chopped
⅓ cup white onion, chopped
2 small serrano peppers, minced
1 Tbsp. lime juice

Blend all ingredients in food processor until smooth. Serve with spelt tortilla chips or brown rice crackers. **Serves 6**.

TIP: *Canned beans are convenient, but it's better to purchase dried beans whenever possible. Soak 1 cup of beans overnight (approximately 8 hours) in 6 to 8 cups clean, pure water. Drain water and follow remaining directions.*

BRUSCHETTA

1 tomato, chopped
½ tsp. balsamic vinegar
¼ tsp. garlic, minced
4 basil leaves, shredded
Sea salt and fresh ground black pepper to taste
4 slices spelt or millet bread

Preheat oven to 375 degrees. Mix tomato, vinegar, and spices. Spoon equal amounts onto bread slices and toast in toaster oven or oven until crisp. **Serves 4**.

TIP: *To increase flavor, refrigerate tomato, vinegar, and spice mixture in airtight glass container for 1 hour before spooning onto bread.*

NACHOS

½ cup brown rice
1 Tbsp. extra-virgin olive oil
1 onion, cut into large chunks
2 cloves garlic, minced
1 zucchini, cut into large chunks
15-oz. can kidney beans
2 cups peeled tomato, chopped in food processor
2 Tbsp. tomato paste
Sea salt and fresh ground pepper to taste
Spelt tortilla chips
1 carrot, grated
Hummus (page 154)

Cook rice according to package directions. While rice is cooking, heat oil in saucepan over medium heat. Sauté onion and garlic until translucent. Add zucchini and continue to sauté until zucchini is tender. Add beans, tomatoes and tomato paste. Simmer for 5 minutes, adding salt and pepper to taste. When rice is done cooking, add to tomato mixture and let sit for 5–10 minutes to absorb flavor. Arrange tortilla chips on plate and spoon rice mixture onto chips. Sprinkle grated carrot and top with large dollops of Hummus. **Serves 2**.

TIP: *For a lighter taste, sauté in vegetable broth instead of olive oil.*

TIP: *Canned beans are convenient, but it's better to purchase dried beans whenever possible. Soak 1 cup of beans overnight (approximately 8 hours) in 6 to 8 cups clean, pure water. Drain water and follow remaining directions.*

PEPITAS (TOASTED PUMPKIN SEEDS)

1 medium pumpkin
½ tsp. sea salt
½ tsp. chili powder (optional)
½ tsp. garlic powder (optional)

Scoop seeds from pumpkin and rinse until all pulp is removed. A medium pumpkin should yield about 1 cup of seeds. Dry seeds and spread on cookie tray. Sprinkle with salt, chili powder, and garlic powder. Toast in 300-degree oven for 45 minutes, stirring every 15 minutes to avoid burning. **Makes about 1 cup.**

TIP: *Eat as a snack or toss in your favorite soup or salad.*

UN-CAVIAR

15-oz. can black-eyed peas, drained and rinsed
¼ cup green onions, finely chopped
¼ cup red bell pepper, seeded and finely chopped
2 cloves garlic, minced
2 Tbsp. extra-virgin olive oil
1 jalapeño pepper, seeded and finely chopped
Sea salt and fresh ground black pepper to taste

Combine all ingredients in airtight glass container, mixing thoroughly. Refrigerate overnight. Serve with sesame crackers or spelt tortilla chips. **Makes 2½ cups.**

TIP: *Refrigerate in airtight glass container for up to 4 days.*

TIP: *Canned beans are convenient, but it's better to purchase dried beans whenever possible. Soak 1 cup of beans overnight (approximately 8 hours) in 6 to 8 cups clean, pure water. Drain water and follow remaining directions.*

VEGGIE PANINI

1 eggplant, thickly sliced
1 tsp. extra-virgin olive oil
Sea salt to taste
1 red bell pepper, seeded and thickly sliced
2 onions, thinly sliced with rings separated
8 slices millet bread
Pesto (page 187)
2 tomatoes, sliced
2 cups spinach, rinsed and dried

Place eggplant slices flat on cookie sheet. Brush with olive oil and sprinkle with salt. Turn over and repeat. Follow same procedure with peppers on separate cookie sheet. Place both cookie sheets in 400-degree oven and roast until eggplant is tender and peppers are slightly blackened. While vegetables are roasting, heat oil in skillet and sauté onions over medium heat until brown. Spread Pesto on bread slices. On 4 slices, layer eggplant, peppers, onions, tomato, and spinach. Top sandwiches with remaining slices of bread. Brown both sides of sandwich in skillet over medium heat. **Serves 4**.

TIP: *For thicker sandwiches, add artichoke hearts or mushrooms.*

TOMATO CUCUMBER RELISH*

1½ cups fresh tomatoes, diced and seeded

1½ cups cucumber, diced

2 tsp. apple cider vinegar

1 Tbsp. extra-virgin olive oil

1 tsp. cracked black pepper

½ tsp. sea salt

½ tsp. granulated garlic

1½ tsp. fresh cilantro, chopped

1½ Tbsp. red onion, finely diced

Mix all ingredients and place in a small bowl. Store leftover relish in a small glass jar for up to 5 days in the refrigerator. **Makes 3 cups.**

CUCUMBERS WITH LIME

1 cucumber, sliced

2 limes, halved

Sea salt to taste

(Peel cucumber, if preferred.) Spread cucumber slices onto serving plates and cover with fresh-squeezed lime juice. Add salt to taste. **Serves 2**.

TIP: *Refrigerate in airtight glass container for up to 3 days.*

VEGGIE-NUT BARS
(Requires advance preparation)

½ cup hulled sunflower seeds

1 cup pecans

1 cup pistachios

½ cup cashews

½ cup tomato juice

7 stems fresh parsley

2 carrots

2 stalks celery

⅓ onion

½ bell pepper
1 clove garlic
1 Tbsp. basil
¼ tsp. chili powder
1 tsp. tarragon
1 tsp. sea salt
1 tsp. cracked black pepper

Place all seeds and nuts in large bowl. Stir in tomato juice and set aside to soak for 4 hours. Puree vegetables, herbs, and undrained seeds and nuts in food processor (adding seeds and nuts last). Shape mixture into bars and place on a cookie sheet. Bake in oven on lowest setting for 6 hours, turning over halfway through cooking time.

PEACH SALSA

4 peaches, peeled and diced
¼ cup currants
¼ cup red onion, diced
Dash cayenne pepper
2 Tbsp. lemon juice

Combine all ingredients. Marinate in airtight glass container in refrigerator for several hours. Serve chilled or warm with spelt tortilla chips or pita quarters. ***Makes 2½ cups.***

TIP: *Substitute peaches with mangos, pineapple, or nectarines.*

FROSTED GRAPES

½ pound red or white grapes, stemmed

Wash grapes and place on baking sheet in freezer for 45 minutes. Remove from freezer for a quick snack or appetizer. Let sit for 2 minutes before serving. ***Serves 4.***

NO-BAKE GRANOLA

2 cups rolled oats
¼ cup millet flour
¼ cup ground flaxseed
1 tsp. cinnamon
Sea salt to taste
2 Tbsp. concentrated orange juice
¼ cup agave nectar

½ tsp. almond extract

Combine dry ingredients. In separate bowl, mix orange juice, agave, and almond extract. Add to oat mixture and stir until thoroughly mixed. Transfer to airtight glass container and refrigerate. No baking needed! *Makes 2½ cups.*

TIP: *Eat granola as a snack, or crumble and use as a topping or breakfast cereal.*

APPLE-WATERMELON SMOOTHIES

8 oz. sugar-free apple juice
2 cups watermelon, diced
½ cup crushed ice (optional)

Blend all ingredients in blender or food processor until smooth. *Serves 2.*

LUNCH RECIPES

CUCUMBER-SPROUT SALAD
(Requires advance preparation)

2–3 large cucumbers, seeded and chopped
2 cups bean sprouts
2 Tbsp. Cajun Spice Mix (page 186)
1 Tbsp. apple cider vinegar
1 Tbsp. garlic, minced
1 tsp. black bean sauce
3–4 cups snow peas
4–5 water chestnuts, chopped

Toss cucumbers and bean sprouts into a large airtight glass container and set aside. Combine Cajun Spice Mix, vinegar, garlic, and black bean sauce to make a dressing. Pour over the veggies, seal container, and shake. Refrigerate for at least 3 hours, shaking occasionally. Toss in snow peas and water chestnuts just before serving. *Serves 6.*

TIP: *For milder flavor, decrease Cajun Spice Mix.*

TOMATO-BEAN SALAD

1–2 tomatoes, sliced
1 medium onion, sliced
2 tsp. basil, chopped

Sea salt and fresh ground black pepper to taste
3 Tbsp. extra-virgin olive oil
1 Tbsp. red wine vinegar
1½ cups canned chickpeas, rinsed and drained

Divide tomato and onion slices; arrange on two serving plates. Sprinkle with basil, salt, and pepper. Set aside. Whisk together oil and vinegar, adding salt and pepper to taste. Pour over chickpeas and lightly toss until well coated, being careful not to mash the chickpeas. Spoon chickpeas onto tomatoes. Serve chilled. ***Serves 2.***

UN-CAESAR SALAD

2–3 cloves garlic, chopped
5 Tbsp. lemon juice
1 Tbsp. capers (with brine)
4 Tbsp. chickpeas (with liquid)
4 Tbsp. extra-virgin olive oil
2 tsp. apple cider or rice vinegar
2 cups romaine lettuce
¼ tsp. ground black pepper
Spelt bread croutons (see tip to make your own)

Blend first six ingredients until chickpeas are broken into small pieces. Pour over lettuce and toss. Top with black pepper, croutons, and additional capers, if desired. ***Serves 2.***

TIP: *Make croutons by cutting slices of spelt, sesame, or millet bread into squares and allowing them to harden in open air.*

QUINOA CRUNCH SALAD

1 cup quinoa, rinsed
6 Tbsp. extra-virgin olive oil
2 Tbsp. apple cider vinegar
1 Tbsp. lemon juice
½ tsp. vegan Worcestershire sauce
1½ tsp. cracked black pepper
¼ cup carrots, shredded
¼ cup zucchini, chopped
¼ cup sesame seeds
¼ cup hulled sunflower seeds
2 stalks green onion, chopped
6 oz. parsley, spinach, or mixed salad greens

Cook quinoa according to package directions and set aside. Mix oil, vinegar, lemon juice, Worcestershire sauce, and pepper to make dressing. In salad bowl, toss all remaining ingredients. Add quinoa to salad and pour dressing over all. Toss until thoroughly coated. Serve warm or chilled. **Serves 6**.

GARBANZO BEAN SALAD*

15-oz. can chickpeas (garbanzo beans), drained and rinsed
1 cup cucumber, chopped
¼ cup onion, chopped
¼ cup tomato, chopped
¼ cup red bell pepper, chopped
1 Tbsp. parsley, chopped
½ cup extra-virgin olive oil
¼ tsp. cracked black pepper
¼ tsp. oregano
Sea salt to taste

Mix all ingredients; toss and chill. **Serves 6**.

TIP: *Canned beans are convenient, but it's better to purchase dried beans whenever possible. Soak 1 cup of beans overnight (approximately 8 hours) in 6 to 8 cups clean, pure water. Drain water and follow remaining directions.*

CUCUMBER AND ONION SALAD

2 Tbsp. extra-virgin olive oil
4 Tbsp. apple cider vinegar
4 cloves garlic, minced
4 Tbsp. parsley, chopped
1 tsp. dry mustard
2 medium cucumbers, thinly sliced
1 large onion, thinly sliced with rings separated

Whisk together oil, vinegar, garlic, parsley, and dry mustard until well blended. Pour over cucumber and onion, and toss until evenly coated. Chill in airtight glass container for 1 hour before serving. **Serves 4**.

TIP: *Refrigerate remaining salad in airtight glass container for up to 3 days.*

GREEK SALAD

32 oz. fresh baby spinach

1 medium red onion, sliced
15-oz. jar of black olives
4 green onions, chopped
4 Roma tomatoes, sliced
Sea salt and fresh ground black pepper to taste

Wash and separate spinach. Slice red onion and separate rings. Toss all ingredients in bowl with Garlic Herb Dressing (page184). **Serves 4.**

QUICK AND TASTY BLACK BEANS

15-oz. can black beans, drained and rinsed
2–3 cloves garlic, minced
1 tsp. oregano
1 tsp. sea salt
1 tsp. crushed red pepper
1 bay leaf
2–3 cups vegetable broth

Simmer all ingredients in medium saucepan until beans are tender but not mushy, approximately 15 minutes. Remove from heat, drain, and serve with Fresh Salsa (page 186). **Serves 2.**

TIP: *Canned beans are convenient, but it's better to purchase dried beans whenever possible. Soak 1 cup of beans overnight (approximately 8 hours) in 6 to 8 cups clean, pure water. Drain water and follow remaining directions.*

MEXICAN RICE*

1 Tbsp. extra-virgin olive oil
1 Tbsp. garlic, chopped
½ cup onion, chopped
1 cup long-grain brown rice
2 cups peeled tomatoes, chopped in food processor
¼ cup cilantro, chopped
½ tsp. cumin
½ tsp. chili powder
½ tsp. cracked black pepper
½ tsp. cayenne pepper
½ tsp. oregano
1¼ cups clean, pure water

Heat olive oil in saucepan and sauté garlic and onions until soft. Add rice and cook until translucent. Add tomatoes, spices, and clean, pure water. Cook for about 45 minutes until rice is tender, adding more water if necessary. Serve with Quick and Tasty Black Beans (page 162) and Fresh Salsa (page 186). **Serves 5**.

INCREDIBLE SUMMER SLAW*

1 cup radicchio, shredded
¾ cup endive, sliced
1 cup fresh tomato, chopped
½ lb. fresh peas
½ small yellow banana chili pepper
⅛ cup fresh cilantro, chopped
½ small cucumber, chopped
¼ cup black olives, sliced
Pinch of sea salt
Pinch of cracked black pepper
1 clove garlic, minced
⅛ tsp. oregano
2 Tbsp. grape seed oil
1 Tbsp. extra-virgin olive oil
1 Tbsp. fresh lemon juice
1½ tsp. apple cider vinegar

Toss all ingredients in a large bowl and serve. **Serves 4**.

RAINBOW FRUIT SALAD

2 bananas, one whole and one sliced
4 Tbsp. orange juice
1 tsp. liquid stevia
1 orange, peeled and divided into segments
1 cup papaya, cubed
2 cups pineapple, cubed

Blend the whole banana with orange juice and stevia. Set aside. Toss fruit together and place in salad bowl or hollowed-out pineapple rind. Pour the banana sauce over the top and serve. **Serves 4**.

TIP: *Add a cup of your favorite fruit such as strawberries, kiwi, grapes, blueberries, etc.*

AVOCADO SALAD*

2 large heads Bibb lettuce
3 large avocados, crushed
3 cups Tomato Cucumber Relish (page 157)
½ cup Pepitas (page 155)
Garlic Herb Dressing (page 184)

Wash and arrange lettuce leaves; top with avocados and relish. Drizzle with dressing and sprinkle with Pepitas. **Serves 4.**

SUMMER GARDEN SALAD*

2 medium tomatoes, chopped
4 oz. steamed green beans, cut into 1-inch pieces
1 head endive, quartered and sliced
¾ cup radicchio, shredded
1 Tbsp. sunflower seeds
1 Tbsp. fresh garlic, minced
1 Tbsp. extra-virgin olive oil
Sea salt and cracked black pepper to taste
1 Tbsp. fresh herbs (parsley, chive, mint), finely minced

Combine all ingredients in large salad bowl. Toss and serve. **Serves 4.**

GRILLED MUSHROOM SALAD

1½ pounds fresh mushrooms
2 Tbsp. extra-virgin olive oil
1 tsp. granulated garlic
1 Tbsp. parsley, chopped
¼ tsp. sea salt
1 tsp. cracked black pepper
1-pound bag of mixed lettuce
1 cup tomatoes

Coat mushrooms in olive oil, garlic, parsley, salt, and pepper; marinate in airtight glass container for 10–20 minutes. Heat broiler and place mushrooms on baking sheet 4 inches from broiler. Cook for 7 minutes or until mushrooms are tender. Do not overcook. Remove from oven and allow to cool slightly. Place mixed lettuce, tomatoes, and mushrooms in salad bowl and toss with Sesame Ginger Dressing (page185). **Serves 4.**

SAUTÉED BABY SPINACH*

1 Tbsp. extra-virgin olive oil
1 Tbsp. fresh garlic, chopped
32 oz. fresh baby spinach
¼ tsp. sea salt
½ tsp. cracked black pepper

Sauté olive oil and garlic in medium saucepan until golden. Reduce heat and add spinach. As spinach starts to wilt, cover pan. When wilted, stir, cover, and remove from heat. Sprinkle with salt and pepper. Serve hot, cold, or at room temperature. **Serves 6**.

PASTA PRIMAVERA*

16 oz. brown rice pasta
1 cup broccoli, chopped
1 cup cauliflower, chopped
1 cup carrots, chopped
2 tsp. extra-virgin olive oil
6 cloves garlic, sliced
3½ cups peeled tomatoes, chopped in food processor
4 basil leaves
1 tsp. cracked black pepper
Sea salt to taste

Cook pasta according to package directions. While pasta is cooking, steam vegetables. Heat oil in saucepan and sauté garlic, but do not brown. Remove pan from heat and add tomatoes. Simmer for 5 minutes, adding basil, pepper and salt. Toss steamed vegetables with cooked pasta and tomato sauce. **Serves 4**.

CLEANSING CABBAGE SALAD

½ head of cabbage, sliced into ¼-inch strips
1 medium beet, shredded
1 medium sweet onion, chopped
Sea salt and fresh ground black pepper to taste

Combine cabbage, beet, and onion in salad bowl. Toss with your choice of Lemon Grape Seed Oil Dressing (page 185) or Garlic Herb Dressing (page 184). **Serves 4**.

TIP: *For a quick dressing alternative, try blending avocado with clean, pure water in a blender until a thin dressing consistency is reached. Pour over salad and toss.*

FIELD GREENS SALAD*

4 oz. mixed field greens
1 avocado
1 carrot, shredded
1 fresh tomato, chopped
1 Tbsp. sunflower seeds
½ cup sunflower sprouts

Mix all ingredients in a salad bowl and toss with your choice of Lemon Grape Seed Oil Dressing (page 185) or Garlic Herb Dressing (page 184). **Serves 4.**

WHIPPED BUTTERNUT SQUASH*

3 butternut squash (about 4½ cups)
Cinnamon to taste

Cut squash in half and steam until tender. Scoop out pulp and mash. Serve with a touch of cinnamon. **Serves 4.**

BROILED TOMATO SANDWICH

2 Tbsp. extra-virgin olive oil
2 Tbsp. balsamic vinegar
½ tsp. parsley, minced
½ tsp. oregano
½ tsp. granulated garlic
2 tomatoes, thickly sliced
4 slices millet bread
Sea salt and fresh ground black pepper to taste

Whisk together olive oil, vinegar, parsley, oregano, and garlic. Place tomato slices in airtight glass container and cover with oil mixture. Marinate in refrigerator for 1 hour, stirring occasionally. When tomatoes have marinated, set oven to broil. Place bread on baking sheet and lightly brush with olive oil. Place marinated tomatoes on bread and sprinkle with salt and pepper. Broil for 4–5 minutes. Serve open faced. **Serves 2.**

CAULIFLOWER-PEA SOUP

¼ cup barley flour
4 tsp. parsley flakes
1 tsp. onion powder
¼ tsp. dill weed

1 tsp. sea salt
Dash of Spanish paprika
½ tsp. sage
½ tsp. thyme
½ tsp. garlic powder
¼ tsp. marjoram
¼ tsp. savory
1¼ cups blanched almonds or cashews
2 cups clean, pure water
4 cups cauliflower
4 cups peas

Grind first eleven ingredients in blender. Add nuts and enough water to blend the mixture into a smooth sauce. Steam cauliflower and peas. Put all ingredients in stockpot, heat, and serve.

BUTTERNUT TOMATO SOUP

1 medium butternut squash, peeled and diced
2 cups rice or almond milk
4 cups tomatoes, diced
Sea salt to taste
Seasonings to taste (your choice of basil, oregano, dill weed,
    coriander, cardamom, sage, or thyme)
¼ cup chopped green onion

Steam squash and transfer half to blender, adding 1 cup milk and 1 cup tomatoes. Blend well and pour into stockpot. Repeat blending process with remaining squash, 1 cup milk and 1 cup tomatoes. When all blended mixture has been transferred to stockpot, stir in remaining tomatoes plus your choice of seasoning; cook until thoroughly heated. Garnish with green onion and serve. **Serves 4.**

HACIENDA PINTO BEANS*
(Requires advance preparation)

1 cup dry beans
1 tsp. extra-virgin olive oil
1 cup onion, chopped
2 cloves garlic, chopped
3 cups clean, pure water
1 cup fresh tomatoes, chopped

¼ cup fresh cilantro, chopped
1 jalapeño, chopped
¼ tsp. crushed red pepper
1½ tsp. cumin
1½ tsp. oregano

Soak beans overnight (approximately 8 hours) in clean, pure water. Drain and rinse. In a stockpot, heat olive oil over medium heat. Add onion and garlic, and sauté lightly. Add water, beans, and remaining ingredients. Simmer for 2 hours. **Serves 5**.

TIP: *For a quick soak, boil beans in clean, pure water for 2 minutes. Remove beans from heat, cover, and soak for 1 hour.*

SWEET POTATO SALAD*

2 sweet potatoes, peeled, cubed
1 Tbsp. extra-virgin olive oil
¼ cup celery, diced
¼ cup pecans, chopped
¼ cup green onion, chopped
¼ cup Mustard Vinaigrette (page 184)

Preheat oven to 400 degrees. Toss cubed sweet potatoes in a bowl with the olive oil. Bake cubed sweet potatoes on a sheet pan in oven until tender but not mushy (approximately 45 minutes). Allow to cool slightly. Chop celery, pecans, and green onions. Place all ingredients in serving bowl. Toss with Mustard Vinaigrette and serve warm or cold. **Serves 4**.

TIP: *This recipe can be served immediately, or prepared and marinated overnight.*

CROCK-POT BEAN SOUP

½ lb. great northern beans, soaked, drained, and rinsed
½ lb. pinto beans, soaked, drained, and rinsed
1 gallon clean, pure water
32 oz. vegetable broth (optional)
1 large onion, chopped
1 large green pepper, chopped
1 clove garlic, pressed
4 cups tomatoes, chopped
4 stalks celery, chopped
Sea salt to taste

½ tsp. savory
½ tsp. marjoram
2 bay leaves

Soak beans overnight in 6 cups water. Drain water and transfer beans to Crock-Pot. Cook beans in 6 cups fresh water for 8 hours in Crock-Pot. Drain cooking water and return beans to Crock-Pot. Add remaining ingredients and 4 cups fresh water (or vegetable broth). Adjust water or broth amount to achieve desired thickness. Cook on low heat until vegetables are tender. Remove bay leaves and serve with Garlic Bread (page 183).

TIP: *For a quick soak, boil beans in clean, pure water for 2 minutes. Remove beans from heat, cover, and soak for 1 hour. Drain water and replace with 6 cups of fresh clean, pure water before cooking in Crock-Pot.*

DINNER RECIPES

VEGETARIAN CHILI*

1 small eggplant, peeled and diced
½ tsp. sea salt
⅓ cup extra-virgin olive oil
1 small yellow onion, diced
1 small green bell pepper, diced
1 small red bell pepper, diced
1½ tsp. garlic, chopped
3½ cups crushed tomatoes with juice
¾ Tbsp. chili powder
1 tsp. oregano
¾ tsp. black pepper
¾ tsp. fennel seed
15-oz. can pinto beans, rinsed and drained
1½ Tbsp. dill
1 tsp. ground cumin
1½ tsp. basil
3 Tbsp. parsley, chopped
15-oz. can chickpeas, rinsed and drained

Place diced eggplant in colander and sprinkle with sea salt. Let stand 1 hour, then pat dry. Heat oil in stockpot. Add eggplant, onion, peppers, and garlic; sauté until tender. Add rest of ingredients and simmer for 45 minutes. **Serves 6**.

TIP: *Canned beans are convenient, but it's better to purchase dried beans whenever possible. Soak 1 cup of beans overnight (approximately 8 hours) in 6 to 8 cups clean, pure water. Drain water and follow remaining directions.*

QUINOA TABOULI*

1½ cup quinoa
2 medium cucumbers, peeled, seeded, and diced
½ cup fresh parsley, chopped
2 Tbsp. lemon juice
1 tsp. garlic, minced
1 Tbsp. extra-virgin olive oil
Sea salt and pepper to taste

Cook quinoa according to package directions. Let cool, and place in large bowl. Add remaining ingredients, mix thoroughly, and chill. **Serves 4**.

ROASTED BELL PEPPERS*

2 pounds bell peppers (yellow, red, and orange), seeded and sliced
½ tsp. oregano
½ tsp. granulated garlic
½ tsp. sea salt
½ tsp. cracked black pepper
¼ tsp. crushed red pepper

Preheat oven to 400 degrees. Line cookie sheet with foil and spray with olive oil. Lay peppers skin side down; spray or brush with oil and season with half of the seasoning. Turn them over and repeat. Roast in oven until skins start to blacken (approximately 20 minutes). Do not turn them. When skin starts to blacken and split, turn off oven and let them sit in the oven for 5 more minutes. Remove from oven. Enclose peppers in foil from pan and seal edges of foil. Allow peppers to steam inside foil until cool enough to touch (approximately 10 minutes). Open foil, peel skin from peppers, and discard skin. Chop peppers and retain juice from steaming. **Serves 4**.

TIP: *Refrigerate for up to 4 days.*

BROCCOLI ITALIAN STYLE*

1 head broccoli
2 Tbsp. extra-virgin olive oil
¼ tsp. granulated garlic
¼ tsp. sea salt
¼ tsp. cracked black pepper
¼ tsp. sesame seeds

Separate broccoli florets and cut stems to about 1½ inches. Steam until cooked to desired tenderness. Remove from steamer and arrange on serving platter. While still hot, drizzle olive oil and sprinkle garlic, salt, black pepper, and sesame seeds over florets. Serve at room temperature. **Serves 4.**

DILL POTATOES

1 pound white or gold potatoes
4 Tbsp. extra-virgin olive oil
1 Tbsp. dried dill
Sea salt and fresh ground pepper to taste

Cut potatoes into 2-inch pieces. In medium saucepan, cover potatoes with clean, pure water and bring to boil. Reduce heat and simmer for 15 minutes or until potatoes are tender. Drain water and return potatoes to pan over low heat. Add oil, dill, salt, and pepper. Cook over low heat for 5 minutes and serve. **Serves 4.**

TIP: *For faster cook time, dice potatoes into 1-inch cubes.*

BLACK BEAN BURGERS

2 15-oz. cans black beans, rinsed and drained
1 cup steel-cut or rolled oats
1 small onion, chopped
1 jalapeño pepper, seeded and finely chopped
1 clove garlic, minced
½ cup cilantro, chopped
¼ cup applesauce
½ tsp. sea salt
⅓ cup spelt breadcrumbs
2 tsp. extra-virgin olive oil

Mash beans and combine with next seven ingredients. Shape into patties. Coat patties with breadcrumbs. Heat oil in skillet. Cook patties over medium-high heat until lightly browned on both sides. **Serves 6**.

TIP: *Serve on millet hamburger buns and top with your choice of lettuce, tomato, onion, pepper rings, guacamole, pico de gallo, salsa, or unsweetened ketchup.*

TIP: *Canned beans are convenient, but it's better to purchase dried beans whenever possible. Soak 2 cups of beans overnight (approximately 8 hours) in 6 to 8 cups clean, pure water. Drain water and follow remaining directions.*

GAZPACHO*

4½ cups tomato juice (read labels)
1½ tsp. cracked black pepper
½ tsp. sea salt
⅛ tsp. cayenne pepper
⅛ cup extra-virgin olive oil
1 cup vegetable broth
1½ tsp. ground cumin
½ tsp. Un-Soy Sauce (page 187)
1 tsp. chili powder
1 tsp. garlic, minced
1 Tbsp. fresh cilantro, chopped (for garnish)
½ cucumber, chopped (for garnish)

Combine all ingredients in food processor and pulse until thoroughly mixed. Place in large bowl and chill for 2 hours. Serve in chilled bowls. Garnish with chopped avocado, celery, cilantro, onions, or any other chopped fresh vegetable of your choosing. Serve with Garlic Bread (page 183). **Serves 6**.

TIP: *Add jalapeño peppers if you like it hot.*

RICE PASTA WITH LENTIL SAUCE

16 oz. brown rice pasta
15-oz. can red lentil beans, drained and rinsed
2 cups tomatoes, chopped
2 Tbsp. tomato paste
2 cups vegetable broth
1 medium onion, chopped
1 green bell pepper, chopped
1 tsp. basil, chopped

Cook pasta according to package directions, making sure not to overcook. While pasta is cooking, simmer remaining ingredients in medium saucepan for 20 minutes. Pour over pasta and serve with Garlic Bread (page 183). **Serves 4**.

TIP: *Canned beans are convenient, but it's better to purchase dried beans whenever possible. Soak 1 cup of beans overnight (approximately 8 hours) in 6 to 8 cups clean, pure water. Drain water and follow remaining directions.*

VEGGIE POT PIE

1 package frozen spinach
Barley Dough (page 182)
2 potatoes, peeled and chopped
3 carrots, chopped
1 stalk celery, chopped
1 small onion, diced
¼ cup green beans, chopped
¼ cup peas
¼ cup zucchini, diced
32 oz. vegetable broth
1 clove garlic, minced
½ tsp. cumin
½ tsp. tarragon
1 Tbsp. arrowroot

Cook spinach according to package directions, drain, and set aside. Roll out barley dough, press into 9-inch pie pan, and crimp edges with fork, if desired. Cook potatoes, carrots, celery, onion, beans, peas, and zucchini until tender. Spoon onto pie shell and set aside. In medium saucepan, simmer vegetable broth, garlic, cumin, and tarragon over low heat. Slowly stir in arrowroot until slightly thickened. Pour over vegetables and top with spinach. Bake in 400-degree oven for 45 minutes until crust is golden brown. **Serves 4**.

GARDEN VARIETY SOUP

1 cup clean, pure water
2 large carrots, sliced
2 medium potatoes, cubed
1 cup green beans, cut into 1-inch lengths
3 stalks celery, sliced
1 cup broccoli, chopped

1 cup green peas
1 large onion, chopped
¼ cup parsley, chopped
1 tsp. garlic powder
Sea salt to taste
2 tsp. basil
2 bay leaves
4 cups tomato juice (check label)

Heat water in stockpot. Add remaining ingredients and simmer about 30 minutes, or until carrots are tender. Remove bay leaves and serve.

TIP: *Try adding a cup of brown rice or barley to soup.*

LEMON-BASIL PASTA TOSSED WITH BROCCOLI AND ZUCCHINI

16 oz. brown rice pasta
1 cup broccoli, chopped
1 cup zucchini, chopped
½ cup vegetable broth
2 Tbsp. basil, chopped
2 Tbsp. lemon juice
½ tsp. cracked black pepper

Cook pasta according to package directions. Drain and transfer to serving bowl. While pasta is cooking, steam broccoli and zucchini (or substitute your favorite vegetables). Transfer steamed vegetables to pasta bowl. Mix remaining ingredients to make dressing. Pour over pasta and vegetables and toss until evenly coated. Serve with Garlic Bread (page 183). *Serves 4.*

TIP: *This lemon-basil sauce may also be used as a salad dressing. Refrigerate leftovers in airtight glass container for up to 3 days.*

ZUCCHINI CARPACIO*

Note: Create each serving individually on a small plate.

2 oz. arugula
1 zucchini, peeled and thinly sliced
3 Tbsp. extra-virgin olive oil
Sea salt and cracked black pepper to taste

Place ½ oz. of arugula in the center of each plate; arrange zucchini slices around arugula, each slice slightly overlapping the other. Drizzle olive oil over arugula and zucchini; sprinkle with pepper and sea salt to taste. Can also be served with Lemon Grape Seed Oil Dressing (page 185) or Garlic Herb Dressing (page 184). **Serves 4**.

BROWN RICE RISOTTO*

1 Tbsp. extra-virgin olive oil
1 Tbsp. garlic, chopped
¼ cup green onions, chopped
1 cup short-grain brown rice
2 cups vegetable broth
⅓ cup frozen peas

In a saucepan, heat olive oil; add chopped garlic and sauté lightly. Add onions and rice; cook until rice is translucent and coated. Heat vegetable broth in a separate pan and add it one cup at a time to the rice until all broth is absorbed. Stir frequently. Add peas with the last cup of broth. When all broth is absorbed, remove mixture from heat and cover for 5 minutes. Do not overcook, or rice will become mushy. Stir and serve. **Serves 4**.

TIP: *For a lighter taste, sauté in vegetable broth instead of olive oil.*

FIVE BEAN SOUP

1 Tbsp. extra-virgin olive oil
1 clove garlic, minced
1 small onion, diced
1 stalk celery, diced
1 medium carrot, diced
1 Tbsp. barley, rinsed
2 cups vegetable broth
1 cup pinto beans, drained and rinsed
1 cup black beans, drained and rinsed
1 cup kidney beans, drained and rinsed
1 cup navy beans, drained and rinsed
1 cup chickpeas, drained and rinsed
1 cup tomatoes, diced
1 bay leaf
¼ tsp. chopped basil
Sea salt to taste

In medium saucepan, heat oil over low to medium heat. Sauté garlic and onion until translucent. Add remaining ingredients in order listed. Cover and simmer about 30 minutes. *Serves 4*.

MEDITERRANEAN PASTA*

16-oz. pkg. brown rice penne pasta
2 Tbsp. extra-virgin olive oil
6 garlic cloves, chopped
3½ cups whole peeled tomatoes, chopped in food processor
½ cup sun-dried tomatoes, chopped with tomatoes in food processor
½ tsp. cracked black pepper
½ cup fresh basil, chopped slightly, loosely packed
¼ tsp. red pepper flakes (optional)
15-oz. jar artichoke hearts, drained, quartered
15-oz. jar black olives, drained, halved
¼ lb. fresh baby spinach
1 Tbsp. pine nuts

Cook pasta according to package directions. While pasta is cooking, heat 1 Tbsp. olive oil in a medium saucepan. Add chopped garlic; sauté lightly, but do not brown. Add tomatoes and pepper, simmering for 10 minutes. Add basil, pepper flakes, artichoke hearts, olives, and spinach; simmer for 10 minutes. Add nuts and reduce heat to low. Pour sauce over pasta in large serving bowl. *Serves 6*.

ITALIAN GREENS

1 Tbsp. extra-virgin olive oil
1 small onion, diced
5 cloves garlic, thinly sliced
1 cup mushrooms, sliced (optional)
1 cup vegetable broth
2 bunches spinach, washed
2 15-oz. cans chickpeas
Sea salt and fresh ground black pepper to taste

Heat oil in saucepan over medium heat. Sauté onion until translucent. Add garlic and mushrooms. Add broth after 2 minutes or when garlic starts to brown. Bring to boil and reduce broth to half cup. Add spinach. Stir, cover, and steam for 5 minutes. Add chickpeas and cover, cooking until completely warmed. Watch closely overcooking will cause spinach to become wilted. *Serves 2*.

TIP: *Substitute spinach with other leafy greens such as kale.*

TIP: *Canned beans are convenient, but it's better to purchase dried beans whenever possible. Soak 2 cups of beans overnight (approximately 8 hours) in 6 to 8 cups clean, pure water. Drain water and follow remaining directions.*

VEGGIE SHEPHERD'S PIE

2 baking potatoes, peeled and chopped
2 cups tomatoes, chopped
3 coriander leaves
½ tsp. cumin seeds
1½ tsp. extra-virgin olive oil
1 zucchini, diced
½ red bell pepper, seeded and diced
½ yellow bell pepper, seeded and diced
1 cup mushrooms, diced
1 stalk celery, chopped
½ cup peas
Sea salt and fresh ground black pepper to taste

Preheat oven to 350 degrees. Boil potatoes for 10–15 minutes. While potatoes are boiling, blend tomatoes, coriander, and cumin in blender or food processor. Heat oil in saucepan over medium heat and sauté zucchini, peppers, mushrooms, celery, and peas until tender. Add tomato mixture and continue to sauté until thick sauce forms (approximately 5 minutes). Spread tomato/vegetable mixture evenly in 13- by 9-inch glass baking dish. Mash boiled potatoes and spread over tomatoes and vegetables. Brush potatoes with olive oil and sprinkle with salt and pepper. Bake in oven for 20 minutes or until potatoes are slightly browned. ***Serves 4***.

TIP: *For a lighter taste, sauté in coconut oil or vegetable broth instead of olive oil.*

SUN-DRIED TOMATO PASTA*

16-oz. package brown rice penne pasta
1 Tbsp. extra-virgin olive oil
2 Tbsp. garlic, chopped
3½ cups whole peeled tomatoes, chopped in food processor
½ cup sun-dried tomatoes, chopped
1 Tbsp. capers (packed in oil)
½ tsp. crushed red pepper
2 tsp. oregano

1 tsp. cracked black pepper
12 black olives, sliced
2 Tbsp. fresh parsley, chopped

Cook pasta according to package directions. While pasta is cooking, heat olive oil in saucepan and sauté garlic until golden brown. Add crushed tomatoes and sun-dried tomatoes; simmer for 5 minutes. Add capers and spices; simmer for 20 minutes. Add olives and parsley. Toss with pasta. **Serves 4**.

TIP: *For a lighter taste, sauté in vegetable broth instead of olive oil.*

COUNTRY CABBAGE SOUP*

3 15-oz. cans stewed tomatoes
3 cans clean, pure water
1 cup onion, chopped
1 cup celery, chopped
1 cup carrots, chopped
1 head cabbage, chopped
1 tsp. sea salt
1 tsp. cracked black pepper
1 tsp. basil
1 tsp. oregano
2 bay leaves
2 Tbsp. garlic, minced

Combine all ingredients in stockpot and bring to a boil. Reduce heat and simmer for 45 minutes. **Serves 8**.

MINESTRONE*

1 Tbsp. extra-virgin olive oil
2 cloves garlic, chopped
1 small onion, chopped
1 celery stalk, chopped (with leaves)
1 cup green cabbage, chopped
2 cups whole tomatoes, chopped in food processor
2 cups clean, pure water (or vegetable broth)
⅛ cup fresh basil, chopped
⅛ cup fresh parsley, chopped
½ tsp. rosemary
⅛ tsp. oregano

1 cup fresh baby spinach
15-oz. can white beans, drained and rinsed
Sea salt and cracked black pepper to taste

Heat olive oil in stockpot, adding garlic, onion, celery, and cabbage. Sauté until vegetables are tender. Add tomatoes, clean, pure water, and spices; simmer for 30 45 minutes. Add spinach and beans. Stir and simmer for 5 minutes until spinach is wilted and soup is thoroughly heated. **Serves 6**.

TIP: *Canned beans are convenient, but it's better to purchase dried beans whenever possible. Soak 1 cup of beans overnight (approximately 8 hours) in 6 to 8 cups clean, pure water. Drain water and follow remaining directions.*

TORTILLA SOUP

2 Tbsp. extra-virgin olive oil
5 cloves garlic, minced
1 green pepper, seeded and diced
1 large onion, diced
32 oz. vegetable broth
2 15-oz. cans black beans, drained and rinsed
1 cup Fresh Salsa (page 186)
1 avocado, peeled and sliced
6 sprigs cilantro
Spelt tortilla chips

Heat oil in large stockpot over medium heat and sauté garlic, peppers, and onion until translucent. Add vegetable broth, beans, and salsa. Bring to a boil. Reduce heat and simmer for 1 hour. Garnish with sliced avocado, cilantro, and tortilla chips. **Serves 6**.

TIP: *Canned beans are convenient, but it's better to purchase dried beans whenever possible. Soak 2 cups of beans overnight (approximately 8 hours) in 6 to 8 cups clean, pure water. Drain water and follow remaining directions.*

BUTTERBEAN SOUP
(Requires advance preparation)

2 cups dried lima beans
1 bunch parsley, chopped
2 Tbsp. basil, chopped
2 Tbsp. chives, chopped
6 cups clean, pure water

Sea salt and pepper to taste

Soak beans overnight (approximately 8 hours) in clean, pure water. Drain water, leaving beans in pot. Boil beans in 6 cups of clean, pure water until they are soft, approximately 40 minutes. Place chopped herbs, beans, and water in blender. Blend until very smooth, adding salt and pepper to taste. Return to pot and season to taste. Reheat and serve with Garlic Bread (page 183). **Serves 4.**

TIP: *For a quick soak, boil beans in clean, pure water for 2 minutes. Remove beans from heat, cover, and soak for 1 hour. Drain water and replace with 6 cups of fresh clean, pure water before boiling beans for soup recipe.*

MUSHROOM BARLEY SOUP

1 onion, chopped
1 stalk celery, chopped
1 clove garlic, minced
½ pound fresh mushrooms
32 oz. vegetable broth
½ cup barley
¼ tsp. sea salt
¼ tsp. granulated garlic
½ tsp. dill
½ tsp. parsley, chopped
1 carrot, chopped

In stockpot, sauté onion, celery, garlic, and mushrooms in some vegetable broth until vegetables are translucent. Stir in remaining vegetable broth, barley, seasonings, and herbs. Bring to a boil. Reduce heat and simmer for 1 hour. Add carrots and simmer for 45 more minutes. **Serves 4.**

BEVERLY'S BLACK BEAN SOUP
(Contributed by Beverly Kurts; requires advance preparation)

16 oz. dried black beans, rinsed and sorted
6–8 cups clean, pure water
32 oz. vegetable broth
4 cups clean, pure water
1 red onion, finely chopped
½ cup carrots, finely chopped (optional)
½ cup short-grain brown rice
15 oz. refried black beans

All-purpose seasoning to taste
Sea salt and fresh ground black pepper to taste
Cayenne pepper to taste
Chili powder to taste (optional)

Soak beans overnight (approximately 8 hours) in 6 to 8 cups clean, pure water. Drain water, leaving beans in pot. Add vegetable broth, water, onion, carrots, rice, and refried black beans. Season to taste with remaining ingredients. Mix well and simmer over low to medium heat for 1 hour. To avoid burning, do not allow soup to boil; stir frequently. **Serves 8.**

. . . .

TIP: *For a quick soak, boil beans in 6–8 cups of clean, pure water for 2 minutes. Remove beans from heat, cover, and soak for 1 hour.*

FAT-BURNING SOUP
(Adapted from *The 21-Day Fast* by Dr. Bob Rodgers)

6 large green onions, diced
2 green peppers, diced
1 bunch celery, chopped
2 28-oz. cans whole tomatoes
1 small head of cabbage, shredded
1 medium white onion, minced
32 oz. organic vegetable stock
2 cups clean, pure water
4 tsp. onion powder
¼ tsp. crushed celery seed
Sea salt and fresh ground black pepper to taste
Curry to taste (optional)
Parsley to taste (optional)

Combine all ingredients in stockpot and simmer until vegetables are tender. **Serves 8.**

. . . .

TIP: *This is a great Crock-Pot recipe.*

LENTIL SOUP*

2 Tbsp. extra-virgin olive oil
2 celery stalks, chopped
1 medium onion, chopped
2 cloves garlic, chopped
6 cups clean, pure water

1½ cups lentils (washed and rinsed thoroughly)
¾ tsp. thyme
¾ tsp. sea salt
¾ tsp. cracked black pepper
¾ cup baby spinach

Heat olive oil in stockpot. Add celery, onion, and garlic; sauté until tender. Add water, lentils, and spices; simmer until the lentils are tender, approximately 1 hour. Add spinach; simmer for 15 minutes. ***Serves 8.***

BREAD RECIPES

SESAME SPELT BREAD*

2½ pounds whole stone-ground spelt flour
¼ cup ground sesame seeds
½ Tbsp. sea salt
4½ cups coconut or rice milk
2 tsp. additive-free baking powder (page 186)
1½ Tbsp. agave nectar (optional)
¼ cup whole sesame seeds

Preheat oven to 350 degrees. In large bowl, combine flour, ground sesame, salt, milk, and baking powder. Knead into dough, and allow to sit in a warm place until dough rises. Punch down and shape into 2 loaves. Place on baking sheet and bake in oven for 1 hour and 20 minutes. Place a pan of shallow water in the bottom of the oven. When loaves come out of the oven, brush with agave nectar and sprinkle with whole sesame seeds. ***Makes 2 loaves.***

BARLEY DOUGH
(FOR BREAD, PIECRUST, PIZZA CRUST, ETC.)

1 cup barley flour
¼ cup extra-virgin olive oil
3 Tbsp. cold clean, pure water
Almond butter (optional)
Agave nectar (optional)

Mix barley flour, olive oil, and water until dough forms. Prepare loaf pan or 9-inch pie pan by lightly brushing with olive oil. Place ball of dough in loaf pan or roll out between two sheets of wax paper for piecrust. Lightly brush top of loaf or edges of piecrust with almond butter or agave nectar, if desired.

TIP: *You can substitute barley with other gluten-free flours, such as chickpea, spelt, sesame, or millet, according to taste. When substituting flours, keep in mind that bean and nut flours taste better with vegetable dishes than they do with fruits or desserts.*

GARLIC BREAD*

8 slices spelt sourdough bread, thinly sliced (¼-inch thick)
¼ tsp. extra-virgin olive oil
⅛ tsp. granulated garlic
⅛ tsp. cracked black pepper
⅛ tsp. oregano
⅛ tsp. crushed red pepper

Place bread slices on a baking sheet. Spray or lightly brush with olive oil, and sprinkle with spices. Place about 4 inches from broiler and broil for about 3–4 minutes until browned. ***Serves 4.***

ALTERNATIVE: *Toast bread with light brushing of olive oil and sprinkle of sea salt. Double recipe amounts for spices, and mix with 2 Tbsp. extra-virgin olive oil in small serving bowl. Dip bread in oil mixture during meal.*

SALAD DRESSINGS, CONDIMENTS, AND EXTRAS

DAN'S FANTASTIC SALAD DRESSING
(Contributed by Dan Colbert)

¼ cup balsamic vinegar
2 Tbsp. Frontier's Mama Garlic seasoning mix
1 clove garlic, minced
Juice from 1 lemon
Pinch of sea salt
2 Tbsp. clean, pure water
⅔ cup extra-virgin olive oil

Pour vinegar in cruet and add ingredients in order listed. Cover cruet and shake until mixed. Refrigerate in airtight glass container. ***Makes 1 cup.***

TIP: *Purchase a Good Seasons salad cruet at the grocery store. It has measurement lines for vinegar, water, and oil on the bottle, and it comes with an airtight lid.*

BALSAMIC VINAIGRETTE

¾ *cup clean, pure water*
¼ *cup balsamic vinegar*
3 *tsp. capers*
2 *tsp. Dijon mustard*
1½ *tsp. dried basil*
1 *Tbsp. parsley, chopped (optional)*

Combine ingredients and refrigerate in airtight glass container. ***Makes 1 cup.***

GARLIC HERB DRESSING*

1 *cup extra-virgin olive oil*
¼ *cup apple cider vinegar*
4 *Tbsp. garlic, minced*
1 *Tbsp. shallots, minced*
3 *fresh basil leaves, minced*
2 *tsp. fresh oregano, minced*
½ *tsp. fresh thyme, minced*
½ *tsp. fresh parsley, minced*
½ *tsp. fresh tarragon, minced*
½ *tsp. fresh mint leaves, minced*
Sea salt and cracked black pepper to taste

Mix all ingredients together in glass measuring cup. Use as a salad dressing or marinade for poultry or fish. If you prefer a creamier texture, then mix ingredients in a blender or small food processor. ***Makes 1¾ cups.***

TIP: *This is a versatile dressing; you may substitute dried herbs for fresh, or use your choice of herbs. You can also use fresh-squeezed lemon juice instead of the vinegar. Add more herbs for a more intense flavor.*

MUSTARD VINAIGRETTE*

1 *clove garlic, minced*
1 *Tbsp. lemon juice*
½ *tsp. mustard powder*
4 *Tbsp. extra-virgin olive oil*

⅛ tsp. dried parsley
⅛ tsp. dried thyme
⅛ tsp. fresh ground pepper
Pinch sea salt to taste

In a small bowl, thoroughly mix together garlic, lemon juice, and mustard powder until mustard powder is dissolved. Slowly whisk in olive oil until all ingredients are thoroughly mixed and mixture begins to thicken. Add parsley, thyme, pepper, and salt; stir. Can be stored in the refrigerator for 2 weeks in a glass jar. *(**Makes enough for 4 servings of Sweet Potato Salad on page 168.**)*

LEMON GRAPE SEED OIL DRESSING*

½ cup grape seed oil
1 cup canola oil
½ cup fresh lemon juice
1 tsp. fresh lemon peel
2 tsp. garlic, chopped
2 Tbsp. shallot, chopped
¼ tsp. white pepper
½ tsp. sea salt

Mix all ingredients in salad dressing cruet or glass measuring cup. If you prefer a creamier texture, mix ingredients in a blender or small food processor. Pour onto your favorite salad. ***Makes 2½ cups**.*

TIP: *Refrigerate in airtight glass container for up to 2 weeks.*

SESAME GINGER DRESSING*

¼ cup sesame oil
¼ cup toasted sesame seeds
1½ cups extra-virgin olive oil
⅓ cup Un-Soy Sauce (page 187)
⅛ cup fresh ginger
⅛ cup fresh garlic, minced
½ Tbsp. crushed red pepper

Mix all ingredients together and place in salad dressing cruet or glass measuring cup. Pour over salad and serve. ***Makes 2½ cups**.*

TIP: *Refrigerate in an airtight glass container for up to two weeks.*

FRESH SALSA

3 cups tomatoes, chopped
1 medium onion, chopped
1 jalapeño pepper, chopped
1 Tbsp. cilantro, chopped
3 Tbsp. parsley, chopped
2 Tbsp. apple cider vinegar

Mix all ingredients until thoroughly blended. Serve with Quick and Tasty Black Beans (page 162). ***Makes 4–5 cups.***

TIP: *Refrigerate in airtight glass container for 3 days.*

QUICK GUACAMOLE*

16 oz. Hass avocado halves (about 4 avocados)
8 oz. Fresh Salsa (page 186)
1 tsp. lemon juice
Sea salt

Crush avocados to desired consistency. Add salsa and lemon juice, and mix. (Can pulse in food processor if desired.) Add sea salt to taste. ***Serves 8.***

ADDITIVE-FREE BAKING POWDER*

⅓ cup baking soda
⅔ cup crème of tartar
⅔ cup arrowroot

Mix all ingredients thoroughly. Store as you would other spices. Use as substitute for baking powder in all recipes. ***Makes 1⅔ cups.***

CAJUN SPICE MIX

¼ to ½ cup sea salt
2 Tbsp. cayenne pepper
¼ cup Spanish paprika
1½ Tbsp. onion powder
1 Tbsp. fresh ground black pepper
1 Tbsp. fresh ground white pepper
2 Tbsp. garlic powder
2 Tbsp. sweet basil
¼ cup chili powder

¼ *tsp. dried thyme*
¼ *tsp. ground mustard*
⅛ *tsp. ground cloves or coriander*

Combine all ingredients and store in airtight glass container in cool, dry place out of direct sunlight for four to six months. ***Makes about 1½ cup**s.*

PESTO

4 cloves garlic
1 cup basil
1 cup spinach
¾ cup extra-virgin olive oil

Combine garlic, basil, and spinach in food processor. Process until semi-smooth. With processor running, add olive oil in continuous stream. ***Makes about 3 cup**s.*

UN-SOY SAUCE (SOY SAUCE SUBSTITUTE)

8 oz. molasses
3 oz. balsamic vinegar
Sugar to taste
Salt to taste

Whisk or blend molasses and vinegar, adding sugar and salt to taste. Refrigerate in an airtight container for 1–2 months. Can be used as a 1:1 substitute for soy sauce or Bragg's Liquid Aminos. ***Makes 1½ cups***.

APPENDIX B

Recommended Nutritional Products

Please mention Dr. Colbert as the referring physician for the companies listed in this appendix.

Divine Health Nutritional Products

1908 Boothe Circle
Longwood, FL 32750
Phone: (407) 331-7007
Web site: www.drcolbert.com
E-mail: info@drcolbert.com

Divine Health Living Food (phytonutrient powder), Divine Health Green Superfood (phytonutrient powder), Divine Health Multivitamin Unisex, Divine Health Multivitamin Powder, R Lipoic Acid, Divine Health CoQ$_{10}$

Integrative Therapeutics, Inc.

9 Monroe Parkway, Suite 250
Lake Oswego, OR 97035
Phone: (800) 931-1709
Fax: (800) 380-8189
Web site: www.integrativeinc.com

Silybin Phytosome, Green Tea Phytosome

Living Fuel

1409 W. Swann Avenue
Tampa, FL 33606
Phone: (866) 580-3835

Super Greens, Super Beryz

Metagenics

Web site: www.drcolbert.meta-ehealth.com

UltraClear Plus, Plain or Berry (balanced rice protein supplement), UltraFlora IB (beneficial bacteria), UltraGlycemX (high-fiber protein supplement)

Premier Research Lab

200 N Mays #120
Round Rock, TX 78664
Phone: (800) 370-3447

DHLA (dihydrolipoic acid)

TheraSauna QCA Spas, Inc.

1021 State Street
Bettendor, IA 52722
Phone: (888) 729-7727
Web sites: www.therasauna.com; www.qcaspas
.com
E-mail: sales@qcaspas.com

Vital Nutrients

45 Kenneth Dooley Drive
Middleton, CT 06457
Phone: (888) 328-9992
Fax: (888) 328-9993
Web site: www.vitalnutrients.net

NAC (N-acetyl cysteine)

NOTES

CHAPTER 1
I LIVE IN A WORLD FILLED WITH TOXINS

1. Jacqueline Krohn, *Natural Detoxification* (Vancouver, BC: Hartley & Marks Publishers, Inc., 1996).

2. Ibid.

3. Chemical Report, U.S. Environmental Protection Agency, http://www .epa.gov/triexplorer/chemical01.htm?year=1993 (accessed May 1, 2006).

4. E. Cranton, *By-Passing By-Pass* (Troutdale, VA: Medex Publishers, 1996), 97.

5. "Ovarian and Breast Cancer," BreastCancer.org, http://www.breastcancer .org/prv_hist_risk_ovarian.html (accessed March 8, 2006). Also, American Cancer Society, "Overview: Prostate Cancer: How Many Men Get Prostate Cancer?" http://www.cancer.org/docroot/CRI/content/CRI_2_2_1X_How_ many_men_get_prostate_cancer_36.asp?sitearea (accessed March 8, 2006).

6. *Harrison's Principles of Internal Medicine*, 12th edition (New York: McGraw-Hill, 1991).

7. Timothy Kiely, David Donaldson, and Arthur Grube, PhD, *Pesticides Industry Sales and Usage: 2000 and 2001 Market Estimates* (Washington DC: United States Environmental Protection Agency, 2004), http://www.epa.gov/ oppbead1/pestsales/01pestsales/market_estimates2001.pdf#search='EPA%20 Kiely%20Donaldson%20Grube%20Pesticides%20Industry%20Sales%20and%20 Usage' (accessed May 1, 2006).

8. G. T. Sterling, et al., "Heath Effects of Phenoxy Herbicides," *Scandinavian Journal of Work Environmental Health* 12 (1986): 161–173.

9. John Lee, et al., "The Kellogg Report: The Impact of Nutrition, Environment and Lifestyle on the Health of Americans," New York Institute of Health Policy and Practice, The Baird College Center, 1989.

10. Phaedra S. Corso, et al., "Cost of Illness in the 1993 Waterborne *Cryptosporidium* Outbreak, Milwaukee, Wisconsin," *Emerging Infectious Diseases* 9(4) (April 2003): 426–431.

11. 22nd Annual Surgeon General's Report on Smoking and Health.

12. "Formaldehyde and Cancer: Questions and Answers," question 4, National Cancer Institute Fact Sheet, http://www.cancer.gov/cancertopics/ factsheet/Risk/formaldehyde#q4 (accessed April 12, 2006).

13. Bertazzi, et al., "Cancer Mortality of Capacitor Manufacturing Workers," *American Journal of Industrial Medicine* 11 (1987): 165–176.

CHAPTER 2
I BATTLE TOXINS WITHIN MY BODY

1. Don Colbert, MD, *The Bible Cure for Candida and Yeast Infections* (Lake Mary, FL: Siloam, 2001).

2. Office of Pollution Prevention and Toxics, "Chemical Summary for

Acetaldehyde," EPA 749-F-94-003a, U.S. Environmental Protection Agency, August 1994, http://www.epa.gov/chemfact/s_acetal.txt (accessed May 1, 2006).

3. International Agency for Research on Cancer, "IARC Monographs on the Evaluation of Carcinogenic Risk of Chemicals to Man," vol. 36, IARC, Lyon, 101–132.

CHAPTER 3
I NEED TO FACE THE TRUTH ABOUT THE AMERICAN DIET

1. "America's Eating Habits: Changes and Consequences," Elizabeth Frazao, editor, *Agriculture Information Bulletin* No. AIB750, May 1999, U.S. Department of Agriculture, http://www.ers.usda.gov/publications/aib750 (accessed May 1, 2006).

2. "The Politics of Sugar: Why Your Government Lies to You About This Disease-Promoting Ingredient," NewsTarget.com, http://www.newstarget.com/z009797.html (accessed March 21, 2006).

3. C. H. Barrows, "Nutrition and Aging: The Time Has Come to Move From Laboratory Research to Clinical Studies," *Geriatrics* 32 (1977): 39.

4. U.S. Department of Health and Human Services and U.S. Department of Agriculture, *Dietary Guidelines for Americans, 2005*, 6th edition (Washington DC: U.S. Government Printing Office, 2005), 24.

5. Don Colbert, MD, *What You Don't Know May Be Killing You* (Lake Mary, FL: Siloam, 2000, 2004).

CHAPTER 4
THERE ARE MANY BENEFITS TO FASTING

1. Don Colbert, MD, *Toxic Relief* (Lake Mary, FL: Siloam, 2001, 2003).

CHAPTER 5
LIVING A HEALTHIER LIFE THROUGH REGULAR FASTING

1. Don Colbert, MD, *The Bible Cure for Diabetes* (Lake Mary, FL: Siloam, 1999).

2. Don Colbert, MD, *The Bible Cure for High Blood Pressure* (Lake Mary, FL: Siloam, 2001).

3. Don Colbert, MD, *The Bible Cure for Colds, Flu and Sinus Infections* (Lake Mary, FL: Siloam, 2004).

CHAPTER 7
SUPPORTING MY LIVER WITH NUTRITION

1. Janet Raloff, "Microwaves Bedevil a B Vitamin—Research Indicates Overcooking and Microwaving Meat and Dairy Foods Inactivate Vitamin B_{12}— Brief Article," *Science News* 153 (February 14, 1998), 105, accessed via http://www.findarticles.com/p/articles/mi_m1200/is_n7_v153/ai_20346932 (accessed February 22, 2006), in "Ask Natural Life…How Safe and Healthy Is Microwave Cooking?," *Natural Life* magazine, May/June 2005, http://www.life.ca/nl/103/microwave.html (accessed February 22, 2006).

2. Ed and Elisa McClure, *Eat Your Way to a Healthy Life* (Lake Mary, FL: Siloam, 2006).

3. Don Colbert, MD, *Deadly Emotions* (Nashville, TN: Thomas Nelson, 2003).

4. D. Conacher, "Troubled Waters on Tap: Organic Chemicals in Public Drinking Water Systems and the Failure of Regulation," Washington DC Center for Study of Responsive Law, 1988: 114.

5. Don Colbert, MD, *The Seven Pillars of Health* (Lake Mary, FL: Siloam, 2007).

6. Kenneth F. Ferraro, "Firm Believers" Religion, Body Weight, and Well-Being," *Review of Religious Research* 39(3) (March 1998): 224ff, referenced in Beth Forbes, "Firm Believers More Likely to Be Flabby, Purdue Study Finds," *Purdue News*, March 1998, http://news.uns.purdue.edu/html14ever/9803.Ferraro.fat.html (accessed February 21, 2006).

7. Bob Rodgers, *The 21-Day Fast* (Louisville, KY: Bob Rodgers Ministries, 2001), 63–67.

8. "Cancer Clusters," Virginia Cancer Registry, Virginia Department of Health, http://www.vahealth.org/cdpc/cancer/cancerclusters.asp (accessed May 5, 2006).

CHAPTER 8
DETOXIFYING MY BODY WITH JUICES

1. "Water = Life's Basic Building Block," Water Pollution, accessed via http://www.bobsilverstein.com/SaveHawaii-WaterPollution.htm (accessed February 3, 2006).

2. Philip Brasher, Associated Press, "One-Quarter of Organic Produce Contains Pesticides, Study Finds" May 8, 2002, Integrated Pest Management, Ohio State University, http://ipm.osu.edu/trans/052_082.htm (accessed February 23, 2006)

3. Environmental Working Group, "Report Card: Pesticides in Produce," *Food News*, http://www.foodnews.org/reportcard.php (accessed April 26, 2006).

4. David J. Hanson, "Administration Seeks Tighter Curbs on Exports of Unregistered Pesticides," *Chemical and Engineering News*, February 14, 1994, 16–17 as cited in "Mexican Use of Unregistered US Pesticides," http://www.american.edu/TED/mexpest.htm (accessed April 26, 2006).

5. Elson M. Haas, MD, *Staying Healthy With Nutrition* (Berkeley, CA: Celestial Arts Pub., 1992).

6. U.S. Department of Health and Human Services and U.S. Department of Agriculture, *Dietary Guidelines for Americans, 2005*.

7. Carol S. Johnston, et al., "More Americans Are Eating '5 A Day' but Intakes of Dark Green and Cruciferous Vegetables Remain Low," *Journal of Nutrition* 130 (December 2000): 3063–3067, http://jn.nutrition.org/cgi/content/full/130/1⅔063 (accessed April 13, 2006).

8. "Vegetables Without Vitamins," *Life Extension Journal*, March 2001, http://www.lef.org/magazine/mag2001/mar2001_report_vegetables.html (accessed February 22, 2006).

9. Don Colbert, MD, *What Would Jesus Eat?* (Nashville, TN: Thomas Nelson, Inc., 2002).

Dr. Don Colbert...
a man on a mission

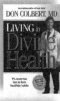

Take healthy action today for a disease-free tomorrow!
You don't have to get cancer or heart disease! In fact, you don't need to be a poor-health statistic at all. Living in Divine Health takes you on a fascinating journey into the world of disease-preventing nutrition.

$9.99 / 1-59185-885-2

Make better health decisions.
You already know that proper diet, exercise, controlling your environment, and rest can keep you in good health. But is that enough? Here is the rest of the story.

$ 9.99 / 1-59185-217-X

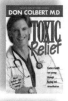

Cleanse your body in 30 days.
Is your body sending you distress signals? Are you overfed and under-nourished? You may be toxic. Now you can detoxify your body right down to the cellular level.

$ 9.99 / 1-59185-213-7

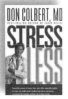

Do you want to live a stress-free life?
Americans are the most stressed people in the world. Dr. Colbert explains why this epidemic of stress is out of control and what to do to regain a peaceful, harmonious life.

$19.99 / 1-59185-611-6

For more information:
Call 407-331-7007
Or visit www.drcolbert.com

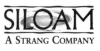

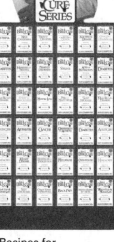

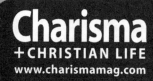